Old Heart Child's Eyes
A Diary of Miracles

Nancy Angel Doetzel, PhD

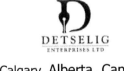

DETSELIG
ENTERPRISES LTD

Calgary, Alberta, Canada

Old Heart Child's Eyes: A Personal Diary

© 2010 Nancy Doetzel

Library and Archives Canada Cataloguing in Publication
Doetzel, Nancy, 1953-
    Old heart, child eyes : a diary of miracles / Nancy Doetzel.

ISBN 978-1-55059-394-5

    1. Doetzel, Nancy, 1953-. 2. Christian biography.
3. Cancer--Patients--Biography. 4. College teachers--Biography.
5. Forgiveness. 6. Spirituality. 7. Self-care, Health. I. Title

BV4501.3.D64 2010   248.092   C2010-902277-7

Detselig Enterprises Ltd.   www.temerondetselig.com
210, 1220 Kensington Rd NW   temeron@telusplanet.net
Calgary, Alberta   Phone: (403) 283-0900
T2N 3P5   Fax: (403) 283-6947

DETSELIG
ENTERPRISES LTD

Detselig Enterprises Ltd. acknowledges the support of
the Government of Canada through the Canada Books
Program for our publishing program

Also acknowledged is the support of the Alberta
Foundation for the Arts for our publishing program.

Cover photo by Ken Doetzel

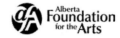

Cover design by Marco Governali

ISBN 978-1-55059-394-5   Printed in Canada

Contents

Introduction

I acknowledge that no two people exist within the exact same reality, or construct duplicate meanings from their individual life experiences. Nobody views an event from an identical stand point, or shares a totally common perspective about life. Each of us embraces our own unique reality and versions of truth. What I share from my writings, within this autoethnography, is based on my own remembered reality, and the meanings I have attached to whatever challenges I faced. I have written this book with a sincere commitment to present insights that I have gained from being a daughter, wife, student, journalist, friend, sister, educator, musician, researcher and cancer survivor. This autoethnograpy is heart centred and expresses my deepest felt truths. I started writing this book after being diagnosed with cancer and informed that I may only have six months to live.

While on my scholarly journey to obtain my PhD, I applied teachings I received when studying to be a social scientist, therapist and educator. I examine my life experiences through the lens of appreciative inquiry, which encourages us to observe a glass as being half full, instead of half empty. I incorporate my newspaper columns, songs and journal entries to reveal some of my life story.

Through my writings I share ways I worked towards honoring my commitment in marriage, forgiving the man who took my brother's life and applying spiritual insights gained from a childhood near-death experience.

This book is dedicated to my family, friends, and teachers who have stood by me during my fight to beat cancer and assisted me in my scholarly journey towards obtaining a PhD. I will be forever grateful for their presence in my life.

It is hoped that this book can assist scholars on a journey towards writing an autoethnograpy or inspire readers to work towards reaching their full potential selves.

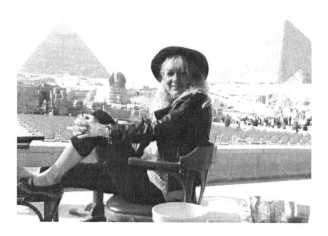

Finding one's full potential self may involve captivating a childlike sense of wonder and passion for life. Embracing the miracle mindedness and grateful heart of a child could enable truth seekers to see a tree within an acorn, a butterfly within a caterpillar, and a rainbow within a storm. As Pascal suggested, the heart has reason that reason doesn't know.

Terry Fox demonstrated miracle mindedness when he stated that "no dream is impossible to achieve" . . . before he set out on his marathon of hope. His intention was to eradicate the suffering of others. When I walked beside him in Thunder Bay, I never anticipated ever losing my father to cancer, or ever being diagnosed with the same disease. While interviewing him, I noticed he spoke from a wise heart. Terry continues to be an inspiration to countless people, including me.

This book is intended to encourage readers to live a healthy, balanced life by taking care of their mind, body and spirit.

1

Loving to Live

Oh God, no! A life threatening illness cannot really be happening to me! There are too many experiences yet to be lived, too many songs unwritten, too many photos not taken, too many friends I haven't met, too many stories untold, too many dances not danced, too much knowledge to be gained, too many students waiting to be taught. I feel like a helpless caterpillar attempting to dodge being trampled on and crushed before spinning a cocoon and ever reaching a full butterfly stage. I am anticipating some kind of divine intervention, to alter my circumstances. I am trying to view my circumstances through child eyes.

I love working as a photographer and reporter for a community newspaper. I am remembering interviewing and spending time with Terry Fox. I am in the commencing stages of completing writing and singing songs for a new CD. I have just finished my university masters thesis and I have been accepted into several doctorate programs. I recently celebrated a major wedding anniversary, on the shores of Lake Superior, with Ken. I am very passionate about life and aspire to live a very long time.

Tears are flooding my face as major clouds burst within my thundering heart. Fragments of my life are flashing before me like lightening casting shadows upon my future. I stair at photos of my father and brother and I feel a tugging-towards-heaven sensation. I question whether or not I am going take a sudden flight on the wings of God's angels to join my brother and dad in heaven. Am I being called to return to my Creator, I ask myself? The thought of leaving some loved ones behind in this world, to unite with other loved ones in heaven, feels like a tug of war between two realms.

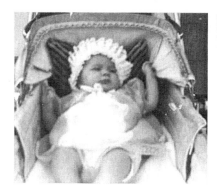 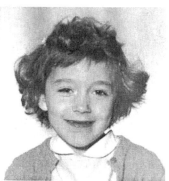

I scan the photographs on my wall reminding me of my childhood days. Pretending not to know what I knew was often a means of survival for me in a world demanding conformity to a set of norms. When not embracing my authenticity, I felt like I wasn't being true to my Creator, to my Irish/Aboriginal culture, to my elders and to myself. Now, I am wondering if I can pretend not to know what I've just

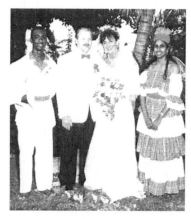 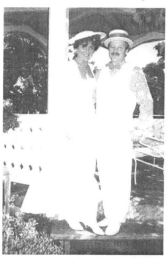

been told about my illness. Can I wash it away, like an ocean wave eradicates footprints in the sand? I question whether or not my nagging passion for living every day to the fullest has been some kind of indicator that my life could be cut shorter than I ever anticipated.

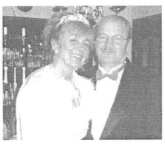

I recall teachings I received about appreciative inquiry. I reflect about the best of what has been and what is. I envision possibilities of the best of what might be. I think about the best of what should be, despite the cancer diagnosis. I apply faith and hope, while envisioning and praying for the best outcome to occur. I foresee myself being healed. This realm of possibility is within me. I believe in miracles.

Disregarding my fear and being courageous means I need to push forward and believe that I am in much larger hands than any doctor's. I need to accept the best of "what is." Watching the waves continuously hitting the shores of Lake Superior has a soothing effect on me, after I leave the clinic.

Communing with nature and being passionate about living has kept my spirit nurtured throughout my life. During my school days, I often strolled through pathways in a forest close to the school, where I admired tall hugging birch trees and ascending rock cuts. In early evenings, I liked to walk to the shores of Lake Superior to savor the fiery orange colors of a sunset. By candlelight at night, I often read adventure books and Biblical passages, and then wrote reflections in my treasured birch-bark diary.

The writings demonstrate my innate yearning to hold an unconditional positive regard for others. I am being taught by whoever I meet, and am willing to listen to. Within my writings, fact and fiction are bound in kind of a sacred discourse. I write intimate letters to my Creator, as a trustworthy friend. My blessings and sorrows are shared in these letters and I often request my Creator's assistance in discernments. Everywhere I go, I carry a diary, as if it is attached to my heart with a sacred golden string. It is usually tucked within my purse, beside my wallet. I believe that someday I may revisit my past experiences, through my writings, and perhaps discover a new version of who I am now, and who I was then, and what my truth has become. I may come to recognize the "strange in the familiar" and the "general in the particular" when I re-read my reflections written in these dairies.

My printed notes etched in a ragged diary, with the title, "Grade 3 Mean kids," tug my heart whenever I read my prose about having received "the ugliest kid award" at age 7. It was recess when my peers saw me relaxing beneath a birch tree on the school grounds. They rushed towards me laughing and then handed me a sketch of a skeleton wearing huge glasses and having one eye double the size of the other. (I was very skinny when in grade three and I did wear "coke bottle" type glasses that magnified one eye in which I had poor vision.) But, when I look back, I can recall that there were also other students who were very thin and wore glasses.

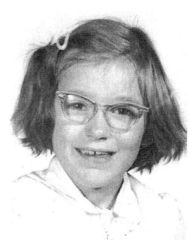

I was known in grade three for having had high marks in spelling, English and math. Thus, students had requested my assistance in studying before tests. I recall running home from school the day I was given the sketch, and weeping endlessly, while in my father's arms. I asked him why kids were so cruel. He told me that I needed to forgive them, because they really were not aware of how hurtful their actions were. He told me to write a poem about my feelings, in my dairy, and then to come watch a humorous television show with him.

My diary, hidden in a trunk, contains many tear-stained pages with inscribed messages I wrote during a lengthy hospital stay. At age ten, I was diagnosed with double pneumonia and spent recovery time in an oxygen tent in a hospital during the Christmas season. I coughed continuously and sometimes at night I would totally lose my ability to breathe. I felt as if someone was strangling me, and when attempting to scream for help, I could not speak. I felt paralyzed and helpless lying in bed in a dungy hospital room, wondering if I would suddenly fall asleep and never wake up again. One evening, I fell into a very deep asleep and then awakened suddenly gasping for air. My lungs seemed to have stopped functioning. I called out to Jesus, and felt as if He was embracing me. Suddenly, a nurse started to pound my back and it seemed as if I was able to breathe again. She mentioned that I had been choking and would need to stay longer in the hospital. I was put into an oxygen tent to enable me to breathe.

On Christmas day, I begged my doctor to allow me to go home for Christmas to be with my family. I stayed up nearly all night long Christmas Eve with my brother and sister and then arose in early morning to open my gifts. During a peak moment of excitement, while ripping open a package containing a warm fuzzy teddy bear, I started to cough and choke and then gasp for air continuously. I could not breathe and my brother and sister yelled that my face was turning blue, as I desperately gasped for air, and appeared to be passing out. I sensed myself suddenly flying around the room, seemingly to have exited from my body, after I was no longer able to breathe. Then, I acknowledged myself looking down at a lifeless self, lying motionless on our green living room carpet, and holding on to my precious teddy bear. I could clearly see and hear my brother and sister screaming, while my mother was speaking to a doctor

11 Loving to Live

on the telephone, and my father was calling out to Jesus, in prayer. I was unable to move or to talk. I could see my dad lifting my limb body from the rug, turning me upside down and pounding on my back. I recall feeling a powerful jolt, as if electricity had struck me, when I heard dad singing "Silent Night." It seemed as if suddenly I was being called away from the arms of Jesus and beckoned back to a lovingly embrace of my dad hugging me. It appeared as if I had awakened from a very haunting emotional dream.

I was soon rushed back to the hospital and was put in an oxygen tent again. My lungs remained congested for several months and I was unable to return to school. I read books, wrote stories in my diary, and made rag dolls, to pass my time away while hospitalized. There were some suspicions at the time that I may have cystic fibrosis. However, I miraculously healed and returned to school after more than six months of being ill. According to my grade five teacher, I was excelling in my studies, and he suggested that I skip a grade. My memory and ability to focus in class appeared to have greatly improved. Like some kind of rights of passage, I had taken on the look of a mature studious learner. In my school bag I always carried a sacred diary, which contained some reflections about my illness, about what I had viewed as a dream and about my experiences of returning to school, after spending months in the hospital.

When I lost one of my treasured birch bark diaries while en route to the Holy Land many years after my lengthy hospital stay, I felt as if a part of my heart had been eradicated. I search and search and pray and pray. I believe that my sacred book may have fallen from one of my carry-on pieces of luggage.

Later, while touring sites where Jesus had wept and prayed, I question whether or not somebody is reading my diary, filled with self revelations. I encounter moments when I feel exposed at the thought of someone entering into my mind and heart through my reflective writings. I wonder whether or not some kind of mystical occurrence had taken place. If so, would my sacred diary suddenly re-appear and miraculously fall into my beckoning hands?

Like a grieving child, I mope around for a few days while continuously searching for my irreplaceable dairy. I telephone airline representatives to ask them to search for my treasure, as if it contained a monetary fortune.

I am despondent when informed that my sacred memoirs probably had been swept up by the cleaners and heaped into a garbage bin before thrown into a dumpster and later burned with other refuse. I want to scream at the airlines representatives, to give voice to my writings. But my heart silences me, with sensitivity towards innocent people just being messengers.

Now is the ideal time for me to start a new page of my diary. It is like experiencing a form of "tabula rasa" (being born with a blank slate) because I feel like my past is being erased and a fresh start is about to commence. An opportunity to let go of some of my painful history is presented. One of my major diaries is gone but so was yesterday. All I have to embrace is the untarnished moment of the present. I observe the sun setting on my past and rising on a fresh tomorrow.

Again, it would be my choice how I would script my tomorrow, construct my reality and what I would enter into a new diary. What I would come to define as real would become real in its consequences. Perhaps at the right time, in the right place, my former diary would re-appear. On the back cover of this dairy, my address and phone number had been engraved within a heart sketch. Beneath that information on the back cover was the Serenity Prayer: "God Grant me the Serenity to Accept the Things I cannot Change . . . the courage to change the things and the wisdom to know the difference." I am hoping that this prayer will assist in bringing my sacred book back to me someday. I often visualize a needy person clutching my dairy and re-connecting with his/her Creator, the God of his/her understanding.

On the cover of a new diary, I wrote:

We teach who we are. Our utterances are interpretive and may not represent an absolute truth. Therefore, I aspire to let my life speak. My life mission is to ignite spirit within whomever the Creator puts on my path. I believe that we may be the only book of wisdom that some people read, so we should be cautious about what our actions signify to others. It is by our actions that we indicate whether or not our intentions are genuinely heart centred. We are both spiritual and human beings, but not in a dualistic way, rather embracing two aspects of a single nature. The ways that we synergize our hearts and minds are our choice, and whatever happens to us, we can elect our reciprocation, which becomes our voice.

I am being reflective of what I wrote on the front cover of my diary and am electing to persevere after being suddenly challenged by an unexpected health crisis. It is a beautiful sunshiny August afternoon, when I sense the voice of my inner child screaming to be heard and beseeching for connection with an empathetic woman, after a physician has announced that my life could be on the line. Like a slap on a new-born baby's behind to induce a human cry, I sense a whack on my psyche with the doctor's disquieting announcement which is an abrupt wake-up call to my existence. Being told that cancer could annihilate my life within a few months, coerces me to look death in the face and hang on to my dear life. During the traumatic moments of hearing about my diagnosis, the voices of three female cancer survivors embrace me, giving me the courage to fight for my life.

These women's gallant voices of survival have a psychological, social and cultural influence on how I perceive my diagnosis and view my ability to beat cancer. As informal teachers, they model attitudes and choices that are helping me to cope with my situation. Their voices are anchors while I stop myself from sinking from the fear of becoming incapacitated by cancer. Their mentored courage is like angel's wings when I am needing to rise above the shock of having to face what I thought would never happen to me.

Several months before I was diagnosed with cancer, I had interviewed Jacki Ralph, lead singer of the Bells. While in the professional role of a news reporter, I had attempted to withhold tears as this famous singer unravelled the story of her painful battles with cancer, while giving me permission to disclose her story in the paper. Jacki explained that she had been diagnosed with cancer on three different occasions and each time she faced surgery and chemotherapy. In the 1990s, Jackie was diagnosed with ovarian cancer and two years after her first diagnosis, she was diagnosed with breast cancer. She had told me that the doctors had diagnosed her three days before her wedding. Then after a brief honeymoon, she went in for surgery and had one breast removed.

When I questioned Jacki about why she appeared to be so joyful despite such health challenges, Jacki said that laughing, smiling and embracing the joys of life helped her to cope with having cancer. She also explained that she had a mission, which gave her a strong sense of purpose. Spurred by her personal experiences with breast cancer, she decided to bring together the distinctive voices of Canada's finest recording artists and record an album to raise funds for the Canadian Cancer Society.

Throughout the interview, I noted Jacki's strength, courage and a drive to beat the disease. Her face radiated as she spoke about her album "In Between Dances" that she had recorded, with other female voices, in aid of cancer research. One of the most powerful statements that she made echoed in my mind, and pumped blood through my heart, as I exited the doctor's office in shock. Jacki had stated that it was her hope and wish that those women with cancer, who are currently in between dances, with flagging spirits and energy, will continue to find the courage to dance.

Coincidently, I had been ballroom dancing in Newport with my husband Ken when two physicians compared some routine tests and discovered that I was experiencing the critical stages of cancer. I was told that unless I had surgery

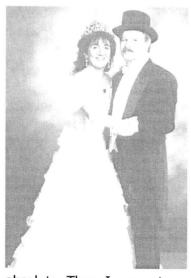

within a few days, I may never dance or sing again. I was in a life or death situation and needed to consent to surgery to enable the doctor to attempt to preserve my life.

After being in university for eight years and receiving three Sociology degrees, I had learned to think critically and to question what the truth was allegedly. I tended to view a diagnosis as a probability, rather than an absolute. Thus, I was not prepared to accept what the doctor had said as being factual. I argued that I felt too healthy to have an illness and I asked the doctor whether the medical profession was just out to receive a financial gain from conducting surgery on me. I recalled having read journal articles that presented countless cases of women receiving unnecessary surgery. I was aware that research findings could not always be accepted as gospel truths because certain variables, such as a passion for life and strong faith may not have been considered as possibly good medicine. These insights led me to question what was being proposed as the only way to save my life. I wondered if a physician was attempting to play God. Could having surgery result in another iatrogenic situation, such as the cases I had researched?

Reflecting on these thoughts brought the voice of Regina, one of my elderly friends, to mind. After Regina had been placed in intensive care, one of her doctors had suggested that she would probably die from cancer or a heart attack soon. Regina asked the doctor if he thought that he was God. She strongly asserted that she'd die when she wanted to or when God wanted her to.

Regina lived to celebrate her 93rd birthday, five years later. For many women, she had mirrored a strong will to live and a determination not to allow an authority figure, such as a physician to take control of her life. After she died, her assertive voice lived on. Strong role models live on in people's hearts.

Marion, a well-known artist, academic and key note speaker also had a strong voice that affected how I viewed her health crisis. When diagnosed with cancer, she had just opened her own art school and was preparing for a run overseas. Before entering chemotherapy, she held a head-shaving ceremony with her friends and went wig shopping. Whenever, she had the energy, she continued to run. After her cancer treatments were finished, she renewed her hopes and dreams by running a 10 K race in Athens and setting up another art school. The disease could not kill her spirit. Like a drop of water in a desert, she gave me major hope.

This hope flowed through my veins the night before my surgery, as I sat at my computer writing a column for the newspaper. I felt an incredible need to have a voice that night and to connect with my community. For many years, people had commented how I had reflected a healthy mind, body and spirit. Now, I wondered if my identity would change when people discovered I had cancer. Until the early morning hours, I sat alone imagining myself being face to face with readers, telling them about my experiences of ballroom dancing and about my incredible journey through the Holy Land. Both experiences had elevated me to a sacred awareness of having had two childhood dreams fulfilled: praying in the Holy Land at places where Jesus had knelt before God and being a Cinderella at a mansion ball.

Reflective question: If you were given six months to live, how would you want to spend your time?

2

Between Dances

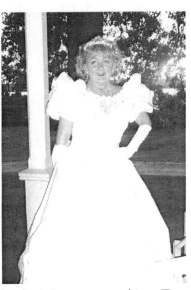

I recall flying high and then landing low when I was ballroom dancing with my husband Ken in Newport, Rhode Island. I had just completed a Masters Degree thesis in Sociology and was anticipating a week of care-free travel. But then, a simple phone message changed my world dramatically, like Cinderella's coach turning back into a pumpkin. Two Thunder Bay doctors were attempting to reach me after I had undergone a routine medical check up, to inform me, not only that I had a life-threatening form of cancer, but that I should return to Thunder Bay immediately.

I thought that this could not really be happening to me.

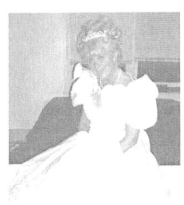

Cancer only happens to other people. The doctors must be making a mistake. I believed that I was too happy and healthy to be ill. My day timer indicated that I was booked solid for the next few years, working on a doctorate, finishing a CD, learning more new dances, making new friends, travelling, etc., etc.

While in a state of shock, I dress in Victorian ball attire and place a sparkling tiara upon my head. My formal silk gloves are stained with tears, when I exit my living quarters, wearing satin dancing slippers and a lacy white gown. "I can finally be Cinderella at a ball," I thought while tripping over a rose bush en route to a beautiful mansion overlooking the ocean.

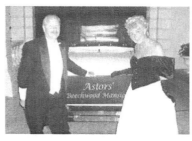

Like Romeo and Juliet, Ken and I savor the light of the moon guiding our steps towards the Newport Mansion. A classical waltz echoing from a ballroom lures us into a romantic mindset, distant from any worries of tomorrow. We embrace one another, as if there may be no tomorrow. Our hearts beat in unison, to the rhythm of a clock about to strike midnight. We wish that we could freeze these sacred moments together and preserve the moonlight.

The clock strikes twelve, the music ends and I look towards the heavens. I pray. I weep. I ask God for courage. I tell Ken that I will return to Newport. I love dancing and am passionate about turning the clock back to the Victorian era.

Upon my dance card, I write down the first few lines of a song titled "Savour the Light of the Moon." I return to my residence and pack my bags to return to Thunder Bay. While on route home, I stare at the heavens reflected from the airplane window and pray for courage. I reflect on my recent visit to the Holy Land and recall having walked where Jesus walked, cried where Jesus cried, and prayed where Jesus prayed. "By His stripes I am healed," I remind myself.

While walking among the wounded, crippled, elderly, multi-cultured and children, I visited sites where Jesus had preached, prayed, performed miracles and suffered greatly. In Bethlehem, I was a guest at the church of Nativity, where Jesus' birth is commemorated and in a mountain desert, I attended a mass where Jesus had shared God's word. At the Jordan River Ken and I had renewed our baptismal promises. I recall when Bishop Henry poured water from the Jordan River on my head; I sensed an overwhelming spiritual awakening.

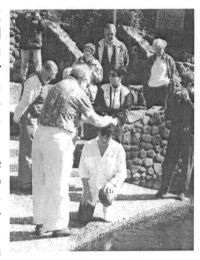

At Cana, close to where Jesus had turned water into wine during a wedding celebration, I had renewed my marriage vows with Ken. Dressed in blue jeans and a denim jacket, I had looked heavenward while immersing myself in the sacredness of these moments. I questioned whether or not I truly existed in an earthly realm.

When visiting the Garden of Gethsemane, Grotto of Betrayal, and church of Agony and Calvary, which were places where Jesus had faced betrayal, mockery, beatings and condemnation, I felt like my heart was being torn open. I cried continuously. I felt as if somebody had stuck a knife through my heart. In my diary I wrote, "it was as if I had stepped inside a Bible and a time machine which took me back to the era when Jesus was being crucified."

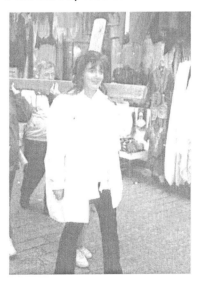

Carrying the cross along the Via Dolorosa, where Jesus had dragged a cross on his fateful journey to the crucifixion, was another heartfelt experience for me. We encountered ridicule, sneers, and heckling. This gave me a tiny fraction of insight into what Jesus encountered en route to Calvary.

Entering the Tomb of the Resurrection was breathtaking for me. I stood in awe, wondering if my whole experience in the Holy Land was just a dream. Candles flickered in the confined space, as if a gentle breeze was passing overhead. I felt an overwhelming sense of peace.

My trip to the Holy Land was a major highlight of that year that I relived and shared in the newspaper column. Other memorable occasions also started flashing through my mind, as I sent my column down cyber space and prayers up towards heaven. When I glanced at the clock, I realized that within a few hours, I would be on an operating table trusting God to guide the physician on how to help preserve my life. My identity seemed to be suddenly transformed into a defenceless tot.

"Could this really be me," I thought, while a priest poured Holy water on my head, blessed me and gave me communion before the surgery. While an orderly, Bill, who was a fellow musician, wheels me on a gurney towards an operating room, I attempt to rise above my circumstances and be connected with my healthier self, by singing an old classic song, "Scarlet Ribbons," as a duet with him. Other patients observing me singing ask me what kind of medication I had been administered. They voice an interest in receiving whatever "happy pills" from their physicians that it appears I have received. I assure them that I have not been given any medicine yet. While laughing at their observations, I am flashing back to when I was viewing the Patch Adams movie, which had a very strong message about laughter being the best medicine. I envision Dr. Adams walking down the hallway with bed pans . . . as his shoes.

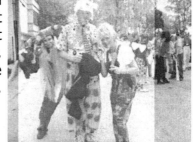

Before the lights go out and my voice is silenced, I feel an incredible sense of inner peace. It is evident to me that people are praying for the physicians to be guided in the surgical process. An hour later, I awake in the hospital recovery room singing a new song that appears to be divinely inspired. I feel a need to voice gratitude for my life, in this song. I ask the nurses for a note pad, and I write down lyrics echoing in my mind. I am still under the influence of whatever medication I was administered before the surgery. I do not have any pain, and I am admiring the bright sunshine and trees swaying outside my window. I am thinking about dancing. I am anticipating becoming a doctor.

My illness has become my teacher and I await new lessons to be learned. There appears to be no individual essence to which I have always remained committed to. I am continuously emerging and being re-formed as I evolve through a life of ever-changing circumstances and relationships. I attract opportunities for continuous learning and for cultivating the process of finding truth. It seems like I am constantly engaging in some kind of observational research that influences my mission to leave this world in better condition than I view it now.

While living life with passion and compassion, I have an innate desire to function as a social scientist: appreciating and supporting human diversity, standing up for others and giving voice to those who have been silenced; and, also acknowledging that anyone I meet has something to teach me, if I am willing to learn. It feels like I had these social values tattooed on my mind and heart, when earning three Sociology degrees, previous to my diagnosis.

I am becoming more insightful about my illness, while listening to stories being told by other patients. A few of them have suggested that I should get my affairs in place, and not embrace a false hope of ever being healed. I have been warned by them that my hair will fall out, if I have chemo therapy. Thus, after getting out of the hospital, I go to a photographer and have many photos taken, with me

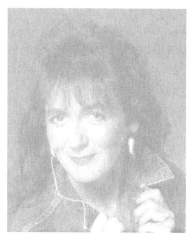

having my long hair. And, I try on some interesting wigs that totally alter my appearance. Having a sense of humor about the thought of possibility becoming bald is one way I am trying to cope with my health situation.

Having fun, despite encountering major challenges in life, has usually involved the two distinct variables of risk and reward. However, I have adopted the belief that keeping sane may depend on propitiating a healthy "madness" within my life, through a creative social means that involves risk. A major risk that I have taken in my life . . . was agreeing to have my life story, using the pseudonym Patches, told in a docu-drama, aired on a cable television station in Thunder Bay, annually for a number of years. I am aware that some observers may view such self disclosure as being a form of madness. I perceive this contracted undertaking as a means of stitching the pieces of my life together to make meaning of challenges I had faced. The project enabled me to reach out to others who may also be searching to find purpose in their pain. Throughout the production, stitching of a heart-shaped patch on a quilt, is underway. The story commences with the sun rising on a person's life and ends with the sun setting on the past. The content is based on diaries of my childhood experiences. An opportunity to honor my father's and brother's lives are given to me, when scripting the docu-drama.

Reflective questions: What are the main memoirs of your childhood that influence your current values, beliefs and aspirations? If you had an opportunity to start a blank slate, how would you choose to begin your new life?

3

Stitching Patches
Born Old to Grow Young

Before I reached age ten, as a young girl born into a Christian family, I had already been referred to as a doctor by my father, Tom boy by my older brother, nurse by my mother, leader by my sister, singer by church goers, future sister by a nun, teacher by teachers and Patches by peers. Despite all these different roles and labels imposed on me, biologically I was just a young Irish/Aboriginal girl aiming for connection with family members, fellow church goers and peers. However, I seemed to be forced to construct a multiple identity that could adapt to the various roles imposed on me by others.

The genesis of a person's self is first represented in youthful activities of game and play. When I was not engaged fishing with the boys, I usually could be found playing the role of a teacher, nun, nurse or singer. During these play periods, I was constructing a personality, influenced by my interaction with others. I was introduced to rules that were associated with each role. My evolving selfhood was influenced by the beliefs, attitudes and expectations of others who were joining in on the activities.

The main social group which gave me a sense of unity of self and a generalized part of my identity as a young child, was my brother's male peer group who allowed me to join them in their fishing trips and football games. I quickly learned the rules of how to dress and the ways to act, in order to be accepted by this male group. I did not dare cry or express fear in the presence of these boys. I appeased them, by collecting worms for their fishing trips, and defending my older brother. While playing football, I became part of an organized process of social activity, as a team member. During the fishing trips, I experienced the competitive venture of who could catch the most or the largest fish.

Another major part of my growing up took place in the formal educational environment of a school and church setting in a small pulp and paper Ontario town. As I strived to become part of a systematic pattern of my social groups, my personality was evolving into a fractional identity, surrounding a limited aspect of my true nature. During grade school, my peers had led me to believe that I was ugly, bony and different and that I appeared "older" than the other children. I was sometimes called Patches with reference to being an unattractive ragamuffin.

At church, however, I was placed into a different role, which was admired and respected by members of a community who shared common beliefs about Jesus. On Sundays, I had the chance to have a voice through singing in a choir and speaking in a Sunday school class that my father taught in a church basement. In this class, dad told us that he knew two major truths: there is a God, and he is not Him. Our weekly assignment involved reading Biblical passages, praying for others and doing good deeds throughout the week. Knowing that dad was the teacher, resulted in me fulfilling class expectations.

At home, dad commonly told me that I was an old soul with a big heart and youthful eyes. He said I would make a major difference in the world, through whatever songs and books I would write. He praised me for the various roles that I was put in a position to play at home. Sometimes, I was expected to 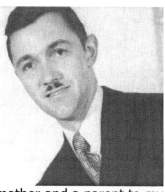 be a doctor and healer to my ill mother and a parent to my sister and brother. Dad often requested that I bring mom some medication and persuade her not to be self destructive. On occasions, mom made errors in which pills she was suppose to swallow and a misjudgment in how many she was prescribed to take. When mom experienced a major mood swing, associated with her illness, I would sometimes leave home for the night, if dad was working midnight shift. At times, I slept under a boat house, close to the shores of Lake Superior or in a local church, or upon some cedar bushes in a nearby forest. When wondering through the bush, meeting a bear never stirred up any fears. I was more afraid of what my mother may do.

Throughout my childhood and teen years, my family represented a significant group who defined my role as being that of a caretaker, in a parental position. Therefore, I possessed a responsible sense of self in relation to other family members. My father and brother insisted that I was becoming a writer and singer, who should aim to record an album and script an autobiography someday. They attempted to reinforce this belief by encouraging me to write in my diary daily and by performing music with me. Based on this relational interaction, a new truth about me began to emerge. I noted that I could break the "don't talk, keep the family secret" rule and thus be given a stronger voice through writing songs and stories. I was commencing a journey towards constructing my full potential self.

I tended to embrace a motherly caretaker's position while caring for drug addicts and alcoholics, who wondered aimlessly and sometimes visited the movie theatre where I worked, as a teenager. Before returning home from work, on one occasion, I had sent an application to a convent hoping that I would be accepted into this religious community, despite being a Protestant. I felt a connection with Nuns, after having been given a voice in theirs and my church and after taking piano lessons from a very caring compassionate Sister, who was tragically killed in a car accident. At my final piano lesson with her, she had told me that I would make a great Nun, and she advised me to consider joining the sisters. My mother laughed when I told her my intention. But, she also reminded me that in my younger years, I had put a bed sheet over my head, as a veil and asked my peers to call me sister.

While being in the presence of the Nuns, I had viewed them as strong, caring compassionate leaders, who truly put their faith into action, while aiming to make a difference in the world. At night, when reading the Bible, I pictured myself as being part of the Sisterhood. I recalled the Sisters having called me "and angel." However, my aspiration to be a Nun was suddenly re-directed by a new relationship with a man who promised to take my hand in marriage within the same year of having met me.

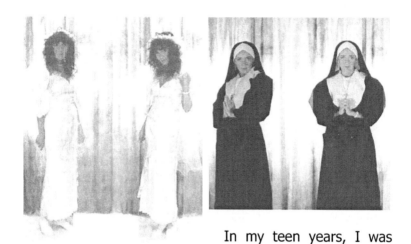

In my teen years, I was forced to make a decision as to whether to pursue the life of a nun, continue to take care of my family, finish high school, or marry Ken, who had pro-posed marriage after only having had a few dates with me. During my decision-making time, I was faced with symp-toms of social saturation and a questioning of my role as a female. I wondered what part of me Ken was interested in marrying. I questioned how somebody, who hardly knew me, could suggest spending the rest of his life with me. I questioned whether or not he was in love with an image of me that he had created, or with the Tom boy, I viewed myself to be. At age seventeen, I was unsure of what the meaning of true romantic love was. However, I felt a connection with this man who listened to me and encouraged me to follow my dreams. Somehow, he had given me a voice and appeared to express an unconditional positive regard for me. When I shared my dreams and aspirations, he suggested that he could assist me in the journey towards fulfilling them.

Without being invited, Ken had shown up at my home one evening when I was with a group of female friends. He said that he was from Saskatchewan, and that "he was a friend of a friend" who had told him that he should meet me. When I answered the door at home, and was met by a long haired bearded man who looked like a biker, I nearly slammed the door in his face. However, somehow when our eyes met, I sensed that he was kind, caring and compassionate. It appeared like we had met sometime, somewhere before. He called me an angel.

Ken had brought a few friends with him to my home, and while they connected with my female friends, Ken and I spent the evening talking about our lives. When I told him that I wanted to be a Nun, he said he had wanted to be a priest, at one time. He claimed that his uncle was a priest and his aunt was a nun. Then, he suggested that he and I should forget pursuing such sacred missions and just get married instead. He insisted that I was his soul mate, who he'd been searching for, and said he would return to my home someday and marry me. At the time, I did not think what was he was saying could be sincere. But, I was proved wrong, when he was true to his word and acted on what he had said. Several times a week, after meeting him, I received letters and phone calls from Saskatchewan.

The third time that Ken proposed marriage to me, I was working at a theatre as a cashier. In my purse, I was carrying one of his sacred love letters. When waiting to serve customers, I would pull his letter from my purse, re-read it and digest his gentle words that entered into and nurtured my heart:

Dear Angel:
I love you Angel, like Jesus loved mankind and he gave up his life to insure us eternity.
Things in life change so fast they are hard to grasp. But Angel, love is God given and I'm sure that no man made force could take or spoil my love for you. I love you Angel more than anything else in this mixed up world. I don't find it at all hard to be true to you. I seemed to have lost interest in things I use to enjoy and I think about love a lot. I don't totally understand what has happened to me, but one thing that I know for sure is that I have found true love and that's all that matters.
    Eternal love, Ken.

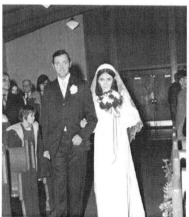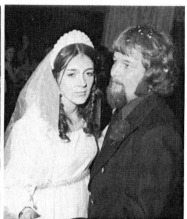

Whenever the telephone rang at the theatre, my heart seemed to skip a beat at the thought that he may be calling me from Saskatchewan. When he did call me one evening, I dumped my box of popcorn, ignored the theatre goers and listened attentively to his third marriage proposal. This time, he had somehow sent a Cupid love arrow through my heart . . . and I responded by saying: "yes, maybe? Yes,"!! "When, where, why, how?"

After thoughts of being married sunk in, I entered a state of shock, left work and jogged to the shores of Lake Superior. There, I meditated in the moonlight and prayed to God to oversee my decision.

The vocabulary used for my wedding vows gave me a romanticist view of myself that carried attributes of personal depth, passion and moral fibre. This perception of myself gave me a sense of inner joy and loyalty. However, my true being was being saturated by peer voices that implied I was an anachronism, not socially constructed properly for the era I was living in. Perhaps this was because I did not aspire to be a mother, and did not dress in the traditional female fashions. Jeans, coveralls and an army jacket were preferred by me, instead of dresses and skirts. Taking correspondence courses about law and journalism, and reading psychology books were my priority over reviewing cook books. And residing in a small shack, once known as a chicken coop, was my choice over living in a traditional classy house. Consequently, I was considered by some other married women to be a radical.

My home community was determined to help me to construct an identity into their ideal of a normal married woman. My high-school principal had requested that I leave school and advised me to learn how to cook, sew and house clean; my peers questioned me about when I would be starting a family. However, since romantic love was at the forefront of my relationship at that time, I had isolated myself from many people outside my family, until I returned to school, as a college student.

Studying radio and television broadcasting at college reinforced a romanticist creative view of self, and gave me a stronger voice in the community. Although I was advised to lower the tone of my speaking voice to sound more masculine on the air waves, I was also given opportunities to write news stories for radio, and television along with the print media. Additionally, I became self expressive when singing classical Irish music at Folklore Festivals, dancing in powwows and modelling high fashion clothing. Connecting with large crowds became a fragmenting and populating self experience that resulted in me becoming somewhat of an extroverted introvert. However, these creative ventures helped me to survive a major heart wrenching crisis in my life.

One evening a major news story, read on the airwaves of the radio station at which I worked, caused me to sense a painful explosion within my heart. I read the tragic news that a former local man and possibly his son had been murdered out west. My intuition kicked in, and I sensed the story had some connection to my life. The following day, I felt as if some of my limbs had been amputated when I realized that the story I had read on the airwaves, with no names released, was a news item about my own brother and his son whose lives had been taken. Many of the good

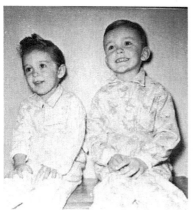

times that I had with my brother Bob flashed through my mind, like time had never passed. I entered into a state of shock, not wanting to believe that this could have really happened to one of my own family members. In the past, the news I had read on the radio or heard about in the media was always about someone else's relatives.

When the Royal Canadian Mounted Police came to my home, I was informed that my brother was rocking his son to sleep and singing to him before he was shot through the head, by a man he'd once believed to be his best friend and mentor. My brother viewed him as a spiritual leader when this man was counterfeiting the ways of Jesus, while preaching brotherhood and love. I recall my brother asking me to send his Bible in the mail, because this friend wanted him to do daily readings. He spoke admirably about him reflecting an angel of light.

This man, charged with taking my brother's life, allegedly had been abusing hallucinogen drugs, previous to the tragic incident. After killing my brother, he stole all his possessions, including his identification, and then burned his body. Evidence presented in court also suggested that my brother's fifteen month old son was later smothered by the same man.

To cope with the emptiness and excruciating pain of experiencing such a loss, I adopted the role of a workaholic. I worked in the helping profession, media and entertainment business. While in the roles of a journalist, singer, model and teacher, I was desperately attempting to persuade the world and myself that I was okay. In each profession, I was being further socialized to be a caretaker, and to follow a set of rules with certain established norms. Again, I became part of a community that was adding to my social structure. While spending time assisting alcoholics to recover, I was aiming to understand the drug culture, to feel more connected with my mother's struggle with prescription drugs, and to better understand the man who took my brother's life, possibly while under the influence of hard drugs. Caring for others distracted me from facing the tragedy of losing my brother, his son and then later . . . losing my father, to cancer.

After receiving news about my brother's death, my father appeared to lose some faith in the goodness of mankind. He became very sad and withdrawn. Hearing that his only son had been murdered shocked and traumatized him. Sometimes, I would observe him holding a photo of my brother on his heart and weeping. He appeared to be losing weight very rapidly. He was demonstrating that his heart had been broken.

As a public school teacher, my father asserted that the only true religion in the world is the religion of love and the solely genuine universal language is the language of the heart. He had learned this model of religion and standpoint about heart language from studying the life of Jesus, his spiritual mentor. A great yearning for light and sacred wisdom led him to investigate Jesus teachings when attending college. He did not refer to Jesus as an exclusive religious leader; he spoke about Jesus' spiritual qualities of unconditional love and how the story of His crucifixion and resurrection had helped him feel hopeful and forgiving during times of tribulation that he faced as an educator. While watching my father battle cancer, I wondered if he was struggling with forgiveness or remaining hopeful that my brother may still show up alive. Would my father's Christian teachings help him to forgive the man who killed his son . . . I wondered?

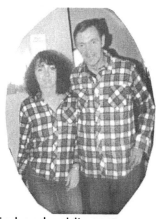

When teaching school, my father had reflected spirituality by giving students novel opportunities for experiential learning. Some students claimed he brought spirit into the classroom when he taught them to sing uplifting songs that he referred to as musical prayers of gratitude. He took them into the forest during science classes, told them how wind and spirit were comparable and encouraged them to respect the wonders of nature as gifts from their Creator. A common assignment he gave to students was for them to check out sunrises, sunsets, and rainbows and then write about them for an English assignment. One of his students who chose to pursue a teaching career referred to him as a wise, caring "man of heart" who manifested spirit and a love for his students and teaching.

This honorable father taught me about spirituality by his peaceful presence, non-judgemental nature, caring compassionate treatment of others, and by his incredible respect for nature. Before cancer resulted in his becoming bedridden, he took me on a meditative walk through a forest when the wind was whistling, and told me the names of all the trees. As he cautiously removed thorns from the stems, while picking a bouquet of wild roses for me, he asked the Creator for forgiveness for removing these beautiful creations from their source of life to express love to his daughter. Then he stared towards the heavens and whistled a joyful Irish melody. I sensed this would be my final venture hand-in-hand in the forest with a loving father I revered as my greatest mentor of spirituality.

During the final hours of my father's life, I embraced his frail body and squeezed his hand while he sang an Irish farewell love song to me. Although by then, he had lost the ability to speak clearly, somehow, miraculously in a song sung from his heart, he revealed to me that my sacred mission in life was to help awaken the inherent latent spirit within anyone the Creator had put into my life. Metaphorically speaking, I was to assist others to evolve from caterpillars into butterflies.

Like my father, I believe that the only true religion is the religion of love and that a solely universal language comes from the heart. When working within the field of addictions, I acknowledged how successful the universal language of the twelve-step Alcoholic Anonymous (AA) program was for helping clients to heal from their addictions. The AA program is based on spiritual principles connected with cultivating self love and love towards others. The twelve steps of AA are comparable to meditative and active spiritual exercises that assist recovering addicts to cultivate spirituality within them.

My involvement in Buddhist meditation practices and Aboriginal powwows have broadened my horizons about how non-Christian religious groups awaken, signify and cultivate spirituality. My sense of spiritual truth is continuously evolving when I acknowledge that the more I learn, the more I realize that I do not know. When I discover "a" fresh truth, this discernment does not indicate that I have found "the" truth.

In hope of gaining some helpful counselling skills and more insight about addicts, I entered into an addictions training/treatment program at a recovery clinic. Viewing the experience as being similar to attending college or university, I was shocked to discover that the learning process involved participating in group therapy, on an equal status to the recovering alcoholics and drug addicts. This enabled a dark curtain to mask my self worth and to internalize a self blaming. I lost my healthy sense of self when isolated from daily relational social experiences and roles. And while being verbally whipped during group therapy by fellow clients and the therapists, making cruel accusations and assumptions, I sensed an inducing of "mental diarrhoea." Their heavy confrontation made me feel like I was being fed ex-lax of the brain to keep the crap flowing. After total immersion into this institutional system for a month, I felt like I had experienced an invasion of the heart. The counsellors and clients applied scare tactics to probe for personal information that invaded my personal spirit.

In mid afternoon, with the others in treatment, I was given the chance to take a walk down to a river, close to the clinic. There, I met a former patient of the clinic, whom had befriended me that year and discouraged me from taking the training program. After having been in treatment at the clinic where I was receiving my training from, John had continued to abuse alcohol and drugs. He had claimed that after he being locked up for a month resulted in him cultivating anger and self hatred. He reminded me that I should not have to be locked up for a month, as I had never abused alcohol or drugs. In an attempt to get me kicked out of the program, he would show up at the clinic, when drunk, and ask the attendant if he could see Angel.

This treatment program was geared to enhance my training to be an addictions counsellor, by putting me through the same treatment process as the alcoholics' and drug addicts' experience of the program. As an institution, the treatment centre had developed its own particular process in terms of values and standards that reinforce ideas of how the world is and the counsellors attempted to impose these values and standards on me.

As part of a twelve step program, I was requested to construct an inventory of my life, by documenting painful memories of major events in my life. I was also expected to seek one-to-one counselling sessions with an alcoholism counsellor and to attend group therapy. During therapy, the counsellors encouraged me to talk about abuse as a child and problems I had encountered. This was like viewing my life backwards.

While immersed in this system, I began to construct a new self image that fit the expectations of the counsellors and clients in treatment. During the training/treatment program, I was continuosly labelled by the counsellors. The structural process of this intense treatment program lead me to develop relationships with others around a limited aspect of my being. To adapt to the relationships I was involved in during group therapy sessions, I identified myself as the daughter of an addict I was advised to do an inventory of my life, which is the 4th step of the AA program. This inventory inspired the scripting of the docu-drama video, "Patches-How Far Can You Run"

I graduated and received an Addictions Counsellor certificate after a total immersion in the training program and passing the exams. On my graduation day, John announced that he had quit using alcohol and drugs and that he never intended to use them again. He said that he had sensed that I had sacrificed my freedom in an attempt to learn how to help alcoholics, like him. Years later John shared his reflections of our friendship during a celebration honoring Ken and I at our wedding anniversary. John stated:

> There have been many occasions that give testimony to the spirit Angel exudes.
> Angel's greatest impact in my life came shortly after I met her.
> Within nine months of our first meeting, I somehow quit drinking alcohol, something others, including myself, consider a miracle. I sobered up after drinking for over seventeen years. I had been drinking very heavy before we met and my life was in a downward spiral. It had become totally unmanageable and without hope. In fact the only thing that kept me going in those days and my sole purpose was worrying about how to get my next

drink. That is, if I wasn't too sick to think about my next drink.

My spiritual awakening back then convinced me that there was something very different about Angel. I have managed to stay sober since I told her that I would never drink alcohol or abuse drugs again. When I made this promise to her I meant it. I have managed to stay clean and sober without attending AA meetings or having a sponsor, which is the route taken by many recovering alcoholics.

Angel's spirit always seemed to affect people. I chuckle silently when I remember how my drinking buddies use to put their drinks down when she entered a bar and how they would whisper "don't bring Angel" when I was invited to a party. Everyone wanted to act well behaved and be good when she was around.

Some people though could not handle Angel's bright light. Perhaps they were confronted by something their own lives lacked and wished they could have her energy and light. But rare are the people that have been so blessed.

Over the years, I have come to know Angel's deep faith and everlasting spirit. I've known her through a lot of trials and tribulations, through her cancer fight and her challenging scholarly journey. Through it all, Angel's faith, hope, love, light and spirit continue to shine.

I expressed a sense of humor when hearing John's appreciative words. I recalled feeling a sense of rejection when I was not invited to certain socials. But, his message led me to realize that I could make a difference by demonstrating compassion towards alcoholics. I had appreciated opportunities to spend time with them and listen to their life stories. I attempted to encourage unemployed males living in the streets to share their stories with others, through disclosure in the media. Sometimes I would write articles about them in the *Thunder Bay Post.*

One afternoon when I arrived at the *Thunder Bay Post* newspaper office, there was a parcel for me from a man whom I had often spoken to when he was living in the streets. He had sent me a photo he'd taken of me singing, along with prose he'd written. There was no return address on the envelope. He wrote:

> To Angel:
> She's all busy with work, school, and stage.
> Driven' by the fire of artistic rage
> Chores done first, then back to the page
> The page of life, filled with music of a caring sage.
> I wish her well, this lady with the haunting voice
> A voice filled with the isolation of the north
> That inner isolation that is not by choice
> But circumstance of the environment, the landscape lonely and disquieted.
> You can hear it in the wind that exhales across the land, a land of angst, melancholy; dispirited; so whatever road she travels, whatever path to come,
> There will always be her gentle feelings for the lost, the broken bum
> She sings not of judgement but of compassion, hope for humanity,
> A true daughter of our northern scene, we know her affectionately as an "angel."
> Sincerely, Bryan

I wept after receiving this very "touching" message of gratitude from Bryan. Then, I searched for him in the streets and at the coffee houses. He had defined me in a different way than I viewed myself. I learned from him how important small altruistic acts of kindness can be to another person. I became aware of how communication from our hearts is a universal language. I realized how valuable and nurturing his message of gratitude was to me. Although this man may no longer be alive, memories of him will exist in my heart eternally. He has been one of my inspirations to "pay it forward" by doing kind acts for at least three other people, after having experienced his thoughtful act. He brought a stronger awareness of how valuable our caring interactions with others can prove to be. Observing his life style enabled me to view my own challenges through a different lens. He showed me a genius within him and helped inspire me to go out on a limb.

Reflective questions: Who could benefit from receiving a message of gratitude from you? How can you "pay it forward" for any acts of kindness you have experienced?

4

Going Out On a Limb

My challenges throughout life have become gems in my learning. I believe that a certain genius within us can appear as a result of our trials and tribulations. A person's wounds and scars can build character. However, many educational and therapeutic institutions tend to view life backwards, rather than focusing on how people with major challenges can excel later in life. Students who have received C's, rather than A's commonly have become very successful and made a major difference in life, by their choices. I have interviewed great artists who claim they had faced major challenges during their youthful years, but later in their lives they had discovered purpose in their pain and had became very famous artists.

Interviewing the famous comedian Red Skelton gave me insight into how his background led him to choose a mission of cheering others up, while retaining his own joy. After revealing a tragic story about a family member, he then stated that "comedy and tragedy can be so close together." He insisted that he was always under the influence of humor. He said he is nice to everyone because man is made

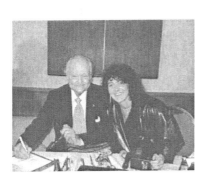
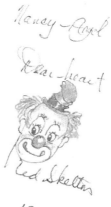

in God's image and the next person he meets may be God. He insisted that laughing is what keeps him from feeling sad or lonesome and that laughter is the best medicine one can ever receive.

Dr. Patch Adams signed himself into a mental institution when he was thinking about commiting suicide. Now, he is a famous medical doctor known for bringing laughter into health care. A famous Country Music artist, Willie Nelson, sings "I'm crazy, but it keeps me from going insane." In an interview, he claimed this song carries a strong message about the importance to taking risks and having fun in life. Going out on a limb, taking risks and going to unsafe places can bring a person into a form of excitement that ignites his or her passion.

The docu-drama video titled, "Patches-How Far Can Your Run" demonstrates an example of how I went out on a limb, took risks and travelled to unsafe places to enable this production to be completed. It is an artistic expression of my reflections about forgiving my mother for her pre-scription drug abuse, and forgiving the man who murdered my brother, for all the grief he caused my family. Patching fragments of my life together within this docu-drama encouraged me to try stepping into my mother's shoes, and also to attempt wearing the moccasins of the man who took my brother's life. A person never really knows how he or she would act, if they had the same circumstances as the individual they are judging. My mother's aggressive behavior toward me, as a child, was often drug induced. The man, who killed my brother, may also have been under the influence of a mind altering drug, and or, also influenced by a satanic following.

The docu-drama brought a part of my father and broth-er back to life, as they were projected upon a movie screen. My mother claimed that her participation in it, was very healing and a celebration of her recovery from perscription drug abuse. My sister appreciated the opportunity to play a clown, which she had actively been throughout her child-hood.

The production gave me a sense of self multiplication by allowing me the capacity to appear to be present in more than one place at a time. Knowing that the docu-drama was being shown on television, in schools and at treatment centres worldwide, gave me a sense of having a strong voice and a global connection.

In addition to the docu-drama's public exposure, my theme song "Patche, How Far Can You Run" was being aired on radio stations across the country. Again, my self image was continuing to emerge according to the ever-changing relationships I faced, after the video and song were released. These creative projects gave me opportunities to connect with others who had faced similar circumstances and were at a point in life where they wanted to forgive someone and let go of their past hurts.

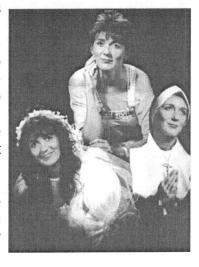

In the docu-drama, the essence of my being, in the role of Patches, evolves to a point of reflecting on how a person's fragmented identity can be stitched together to create a rich multicolored selfhood. My evolved selfhood, which is the freedom to have my own story, leaned on a capacity to express myself publically.

When searching for other female authors, I noted that only a small number of women had written honest autobiographies. And, when women wrote autobiographies, they often used male pseudonyms. This strategy, when writing autobiographical material, enabled them to retain their own identities as scholars, while creating alter egos. Like other female auto biographers, when I scripted my life story, I felt safer using a pseudonym than my own name when referring to self in the docu-drama, as Patches. The name

Patches also suggested gender neutrality. Scripting an auto-biographical docu-drama had helped me acknowledge how the construction of my identity had been influenced by my family, education, life experiences, media, peers and role models.

When the docu-drama was being aired on local television, I felt transparent, knowing that countless people could tune into my life story and assume they knew me. When some viewers referred to me as a "celebrity, movie star, singer or author," I felt like they were piling bricks on my shoulders, and I longed to return to the simple role of a humble student, embracing a text book. Or, alternatively, I was tempted to leave the country and become totally anonymous.

After presenting the docu-drama to some Lakehead University classes, I was encouraged by professors and students to return to that institution and continue pursuing a degree. Within a few months of the drama's public release, I was accepted into another degree program. Soon, I had started to view myself as a scholar hungering for more knowledge. I truly felt humbled, knowing that the more I learned, the more I realized how much I did not know.

During breaks from teaching or taking classes, I spent time off campus at a recording studio, singing original songs and doing freelance reporting for a community newspaper. In a *Thunder Bay Post* feature story, I reported about my parachuting experience to help raise funds for the local hospital.

> The best cure for my anxiety Sunday afternoon before I jumped from 11 000 feet up in the air out of an airplane, was prayer. As I stepped out on to the ledge of the plane, preparing to parachute, I confessed my absolute dependence on God. Before I jumped, I was advised to just let go of the wing, hold my harness and kick up my feet. Full of wonder and excitement, I fell freely through the air, with awe. The wind was blowing at a high speed and the sun sparkled through the clouds. At times I was chilled and breathless. At an alti-

tude of 6000 feet, the parachute chord was pulled and a whole new experience began after having had 30 seconds of freefall. I seemed to be gliding beneath the canopy, and I could appreciate the beauty of the lakes and trees below me. As I steered towards the Candy Mountain air strip, I did a few spins in the air, then landed on the ground several feet from where my husband was standing. I was later informed that I had received an A+ rating on my sky dive and I was thanked for assisting to raise $18 000 for the Thunder Bay Regional Hospital Paediatric Unit.

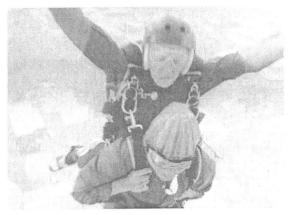

Having successfully parachuted with an intention of altruism truly assisted me to rise above some trying times. I embraced a strong memory of feeling close to God, while free falling from what felt like heaven. I was able to look upward and downward, while catching my breath and praying for a safe landing. I really believed strongly that the arms of God were holding me. The same sensation came over me, when I stepped into a court room in Vancouver.

In the commencement of a new fall semester, I took time out from university classes, to attend the court trial for the man convicted for killing my brother. I cringed and felt knives in my heart when the accused walked into the courtroom, restrained by chains and accompanied by four RCMP officers. He stood about six foot four, was bald, and had a lump on his forehead. He pointed his fingers at the judge and said that Satan was in charge, and would take care of things in the courtroom.

Sitting through the trial felt like having my heart put through a paper shredder. Sometimes, I just wanted to scream or run across the court room and grab the accused by his neck. However, while studying at the university, I had learned some techniques to manage my emotions. Also, a few years before the trial, I had walked on hot coals, without burning my feet, so I believed I could walk through this situation, without getting hurt.

When in the court room, listening to the witnesses unravel horror stories about how my brother had been abused by the accused, I reflected about the experience of walking on hot coals, that I had written about in the *Thunder Bay Post.*

> To walk on a bed of fiery coals was never a goal that I embraced in life. However, stepping beyond fear had been an ongoing aim of my daily existence. And to succeed in spite of any obstacle that may stand in my way, is a major aspiration. Perhaps that is why I was persuaded to venture towards doing a fire walk. I haven't been able to recall an experience that totally compares with walking on a bed of fiery coals. It appeared to be some kind of mini-miracle that reminded me that fear can be changed into joy and celebration when one chooses to leap beyond its apprehensions. Somehow, I'd come to believe that my only reason for being there was to play the journalist's role of observing and taking notes and photographs. On my note pad I had written that the 'four steps to make your performance unlimited are clarity, intent, strategy and action. One is not to be arrogant, nonchalant or motivated by peer pressure, if they choose to do the walk. They must act intuitively, look upward and visualize themselves on the other side of the fire. As one walks across the coals, he or she must think about staying cool.
>
> After reviewing my notes, I got caught up in the spirit. A drum was beating and the crowd was cheering as participants stood in a circle around the coals. I could feel the heat of the coals and was continuously informed of

how fantastic the experience was. Suddenly, I found myself walking barefoot across the coals. I did not burn my feet and I don't recall feeling the heat as I walked. But I'll never forget how exalted I felt when I reached the end of the coals.

During the trial, a crown attorney advised me against showing any emotion in the court room. I was informed that if I cried or expressed my anger, I may influence the jury and the case could be thrown out of court. This meant that the man who allegedly murdered my brother had a voice in court, but I, the survivor was requested to be muted. During the trial, I attempted to cover up any emotions, by hiding my face in my jacket sleeve and muffling the sounds of my tears. I observed the crown examining a possible intention and context of the case, from the accused point of view. According to evidence presented, it appeared as if my brother had refused to participate in some satanic rituals that were initiated by the accused. Thus, for exercising his morals, my brother had been beaten on many occasions by the accused and deprived of food and shelter for him and his son, on freezing cold winter nights. It was stated in court that my brother was limping a lot and he had looked like a skeleton from lack of nourishment. Apparently, the accused had attempted to end my brother's life through continuous abuse, before putting a gun to his head.

The trial ended when the accused was given life in prison as a consequence of taking the life of my brother. When reporters asked me if I believed in capital punishment, I reminded them that killing another human being would not bring my brother or nephew back to life. I later reflected on Jesus' sacred words when He was hanging on a cross and taking his final breaths. Jesus had cried "Father . . . forgive them, for they know not what they do." I sensed that these words were carved on my heart and I believed that I needed to forgive the accused for taking the life of my brother. Forgiving would be practising the sociological teachings of having "quality of mind" and debunking surface evidence. Somehow, from deep within my heart, I felt compassion for this fragmented man who may never had felt loved by his only parents and may have suffered from a scarred heart. Perhaps he had faced anomie and lacked having a value system of any set norms.

Cultivating a skill of applying "sociological imagination" assisted me to reflect upon the relationship between his personal life and how society may have influenced his choices. I could sense towards the end of the trial that my emotions had shifted from anger and resentment into empathy and acceptance. I recalled having been informed about how the accused had lived a life filled with lots of abuse. I tried sympathetic introspection to step into his moccasins, again, just for a few moments. Perhaps, if I lived the same life as he did, my values and beliefs may reflect his. When he pulled the trigger on the gun, he may have believed he was sending my brother off to a better place. It appeared that he could not accept the forgiveness my brother was able to express towards him, in spite of continuous abuse by this man.

When I returned home after attending this trial, I became involved in anti-violence campaigns and attempted to assist others who were facing grief from the loss of family members. I became a victim's rights advocate. Within a year of having attended this trial, I was encouraged by members of my community to run for a seat in the municipal election. They pointed out that this was a special year because I would be studying leadership for my Masters' degree and would be celebrating a special wedding anniversary.

Reflective questions: If you could know that a significant other would be suddenly killed or die, how would you treat this person?

If you could debunk a tragic situation, or wear the shoes of someone you resent . . . would you be able to forgive him or her?

5

The Wings of My Dreams

My husband Ken and I were dressed in white wedding attire when we stepped off a boat at Marina Park in Thunder Bay on a sunshiny July afternoon, to engage in a special wedding anniversary celebration off the shores of Lake Superior. Seagulls were flying overhead, a band was playing the wedding march and crowds were assembled beside a historical train station to watch this unique anniversary ceremony. A cultural flavor was added with Aboriginal, Irish and German dancers. The Town Crier 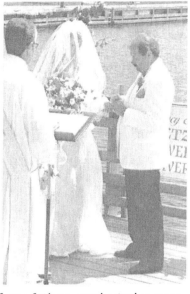 introduced us and a friend of my father conducted a ceremony. To my husband, I sang original love ballads from my new album titled "True Love's A Miracle."

The completion and arrival of the album was a miracle in itself. The recording company had made an error in the address to forward the albums. Apparently they had addressed the package to go to North Bay, instead of Thunder Bay. However, miraculously one box arrived in Thunder Bay at a drop off depot, without any explanation. I received a phone call because my name was on the package. Later, the recording company could not explain how the package of tapes, with the exact number I needed for the celebration, had managed to arrive in Thunder Bay, the day I required them.

"Soon be Together" was one of the songs on the album that I sang at the celebration:

Verse 1
When spring filled the air,
you came from somewhere,
Walked into my life,
called me your future wife,
I was seventeen,
Not sure what love did mean;
wore braids in my hair,
Ragged jeans with a tear.

Chorus:
Though you lived far away,
your letters all did say
We'll soon be together,
I'll love you darling forever.

Verse 2
I laughed when you first said,
someday we'd be wed,
You'd live a happy life
with me as your wife.
You were young,
when you called and asked me,
To marry you that year,
so I could be near.

Verse 3
When you travel away,
your messages still say,
We'll soon be together;
I'll love my bride forever.

This anniversary ceremony had been introduced in the community as part of the summer harborfest activities which continued after sunset. At dusk, I walked barefoot on the Marina boardwalks overlooking Lake Superior shores, to observe the festival fireworks. Watching diamonds sparkling throughout the moonlit sky, while I was dressed in a wedding gown, and standing on the shores of Lake Superior, was sacred for me. Ken and I danced and danced . . . and danced. The wings of our dreams were in motion.

After celebrating this special anniversary and completing three university degrees, I was advised that fall was an ideal time for me to take another risk. In October, I put my hat in the ring as a female candidate for the municipal election, a few hours before the deadline. I was aiming to make a difference and be a voice for the people. While campaigning, I was told Thunder Bay needed grandfather figures on city council. A number of voters said that I was too young to be a candidate and others commented that a woman would not be tough enough to deal with certain city issues. People also reminded me that the position I sought was for an "alderman," not an "alderwoman."

Although I did not win the election, in the context of gaining a seat on council, I was given a stronger voice in my community and the number of votes I received exceeded my expectations. Additionally, I had the chance to see how some of the theory presented in my thesis, titled "Women In Leadership in Health Care and Education" could be applied to real life situations. Running for the election was a learning experience that exceeded what I could have acquired in textbooks or a classroom. This type of experiential learning gave me a voice, a sense of connection with the community, and a drive to continue my education.

My "voice" and ways to connect with others altered as I increased my informal and formal education. Throughout my life, it is obvious that my gender and selfhood were being constructed and reconstructed. When I associated with males, I often adopted a masculine dress code and behavior patterns. However, when I was modelling high fashion outfits or singing on stage with females, my clothes and mannerisms were very feminine. Thus, I noted that although a person's sex is a genetic biological division that separates females and males, his/her gender is that which is perceived as feminine or masculine by the common world
.

Conducting research for my Masters thesis, encouraged me to examine the construction of my gender and introduced me to the empowerment of a feminist lens. By examining life with a fresh lens, I noticed spaces where women had been excluded from the development of knowledge. I also noted that certain characteristics of gender, which I had been taught to accept as natural, were really constructed from false assumptions. By applying a new lens, I began viewing the world from the standpoint of being female. Despite what I had been taught by educational, religious or other social institutions, I could change my lenses to gain new perspectives on life.

The value of the experiential in the acquisition of knowledge became evident to me. By presenting a model or giving evidence of something, people can view what is possible. What other people accomplish can provide a strong motivation for human progress. People tend to learn first with substantial things and then progress to abstractions. Therefore, I believe that learning should present direct application and illustration to build people's interest and then give them a chance to accomplish something. Entering into a training/treatment program and running for an election could be perceived as methods of acquiring knowledge, experientially.

In the absence of knowledge, people tend to act on distorted thinking, affecting the development of their self perception. People may benefit by being put through some kind of process by which they would have the kinks removed from their minds and get rid of nonsense. Preserving old mind sets, as a result of a lack of knowledge, often leads people to undermine their capabilities for reaching their full potential.

I am aiming to move beyond any nonsense and old mind sets that I had cultivated throughout my life. I am now going to enter into an Educational doctoral program at the University of Calgary. I have decided not to pursue a doctorate at the University of Toronto or McMaster University in Hamilton.

Reflective questions: What experiences did you have in life that changed the way you view the world?

How do you view the world differently now?

6

Forever Learning, Forever Dancing

Fear of the unfamiliar caused me to feel paralyzed when I stepped onto the University of Calgary campus for the first time. This university appeared huge and threatening to a graduate student who had adapted to attending classes on a small university campus in Thunder Bay. However, I transcended my fears and chose to enter into a doctorate program after being formally accepted as a PhD student, by the University of Calgary. That year, another new page in my diary had been opened.

During Stampede in July, I spent a week in Calgary to attend the Leadership Institute at the University of Calgary. There, I met two students who believed music could augment certain teachings and they encouraged me to sing a country song with them during a class presentation addressing "bringing joy into the workplace." On the final day of the course, I conformed to the Stampede dress code by wearing cowboy boots, a denim skirt, frilly blouse and cowboy hat to the university class. After class had ended, I hopped on to the C-Train and headed to the Stampede grounds. While reflecting about having to return to Thunder Bay the next day for an MRI medical test to check out whether or not I had a brain tumor, I prayed for an opportunity to meet a new friend to share laughter and dance with at the Stampede.

The stampede grounds were packed when I arrived, but I located a place to relax and read a text book. Sitting alone on a bar stool at an abandoned table may have been an open invitation for others to join me. I was reviewing a book about spiritual leadership when a young Aboriginal man, Don, approached me and asked whether or not I was an angel. He insisted that he saw a bright light framing my face. I asked him what he had been drinking. Then, I questioned this man, dressed in denim jeans and a jacket, how he knew that my nickname was Angel.

Don assured me that he was just looking for someone to talk and laugh with. But his conversation centred on his concerns about his over indulgence in alcohol and hard drugs. He said that he wanted to change his lifestyle and start returning to being a prayerful person. He confided in me that he had recently overdosed on drugs and said he did not want that incident to be repeated. I was wondering why he trusted me with such personal information.

After talking to him about some Christian and Aboriginal teachings in the book I happened to be reading that evening,, he asked me if I would pray for him. I responded by requesting that he also pray for me. So, suddenly two strangers were praying together, inconspicuously, in a bar, at a stampede with country music playing in the background.

As the evening progressed, we danced and laughed about simple things, as if we were siblings, being reunited. Our time together ended after we had watched fireworks illuminate the skies above the stampede grounds. Before parting, I promised Don that if he gave up abusing drugs and alcohol by his upcoming birthday, which was a few months away, I would take him out for dinner to celebrate. I told him that he had a physical resemblance to my late brother Bob, and asked if he would like to become an adopted brother.

At 6 a.m., the following day, I was on a flight back to Thunder Bay where I was booked at the hospital for an MRI test. When I walked into the hospital, I was carrying a camera and a note pad. I suggested to the nurse who was administering the test that I was at the hospital to investigate the process of an MRI test. I assured the nurse that I was healthy, so the test would not show any abnormalities, despite medical suspicions.

After the nurse took a photograph of me sitting on the MRI machine and asked me a few questions, the medical testing commenced. I was given ear plugs and placed in what felt like a miniature submarine. The crashing sounds of the machine gave the sensation of a hammer pounding close to my head. I felt claustrophobic and confined. Within a half hour, the testing was complete and I left the hospital with a friend who took me for brunch at Marina Park. While listening to the Superior waves rush upon the rocky shores, I prayed I would remain healthy. I was excited about playing a major role in a play that evening.

The play was like a final exam for the acting course I was registered in. I was cast in the role of a grade nine student attempting to be queen of the high school prom. When acting on stage, I totally forgot about any health challenges and was diverted from my scholarly role. The experience of being in a stage character assisted me to live fully in the moment and savor joy. Thus, I accepted other opportunities to take the stage. Within the next two weeks, I sang the Messiah with the Thunder Bay Symphony Orchestra choir, performed Liturgical dance during a Mass and modelled white satin gowns for a wedding fashion show. Again, I felt fully present and existing in the now. I had a sense of purpose that transcended any physical discomfort. Thus, to help retain this strong sense of purpose, and feel fully alive, I accepted additional public performance opportunities.

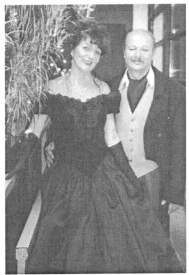

Before returning to my studies in Calgary, my husband Ken and I auditioned to dance in a presentation of the Nutcracker at the Thunder Bay Community Auditorium. After being accepted, we invested long hours into rehearsals. Being amongst a cast of one hundred during the festive season was a chance of a lifetime for us. In a *Thunder Bay Post* newspaper column, I wrote about my experience of dancing in the Nutcracker:

Twas an hour before stage call when all though the community auditorium greenroom, a cast of 100 for the production of the Nutcracker waited patiently for the curtain to rise. After having auditioned in the summer and rehearsed long hours since the fall, we were ready to demonstrate to our incredible artistic director and choreographer, Gina Almgren, that we could make her vision of the Nutcracker a reality. This would be our Christmas gift to such a well-deserving leader who paced the floor in her Grinch slippers throughout the production. While we counted down, a seamstress was still stitching ripped costumes, hairdressers were styling hair, some ballet dancers were massaging their strained muscles and a black cat was being coached on how to enter a basket. A number of the dancers were grabbing a quick snack and stretching before changing into their costumes.

As a cast member, I was hoping that the audience would not notice that I had a triple lip and a double chin, after having experienced a sudden fall on the pavement when I was ill and struggling with balance. I was very grateful for a miraculous makeup job done on my face, before the performance and also for the seamstress' quick hemming of my gown, which probably prevented me from tripping when I waltzed with my husband during the party scene. By the time that the clock had struck seven, the party scene cast was on both sides of the stage, awaiting music cues from the Thunder Bay Symphony Orchestra. I could feel my heart rate increase, as I moved closer to the curtain, holding my husband's hand. This was the first time that we would be on stage together. At that moment, I felt like a vulnerable toddler again. Our fellow cast members were smiling, knowing their sense of merriment would be picked up by the audience.

One of the first cast members to step on stage attempted to mask her disappointment when the black cat in her basket refused to cooperate. The children in the cast appeared to be amused by the cat's unwillingness to participate. Juoini and Deborah Kraft, a husband and wife team who played Mr. and Mrs. Silverhaus, carried the same friendly welcoming approach off stage as they did in their roles. When I asked John Raferty, cast as Drosselmeier, to magically heal my wounded face, he reminded me that being a magician was just an act staged for the Nutcracker.

After the party scene on stage was finished, a huge prop change was taking place behind the scenes to prepare for the battle scene. Suddenly cannons were going off, and Drosselmeir was performing a magic act to enable a tree to grow. Phil Contardo, cast as the Nutcracker, was lying behind the tree, while it was being wheeled off stage. Observing the number of talented Thunder Bay dancers and actors behind the scenes made me feel proud to be part of such a rich community. There was a special energy created when we came together in the production to help make a dream become a reality.

After dancing in the production of the Nutcracker, I launched a CD titled Savour the Light of the Moon, as part of a fundraiser for Cancer Research Foundation and the Thunder Bay Regional Hospital Foundation. The candlelight benefit, which was held on the date of my wedding anniversary, featured Daylin, an International

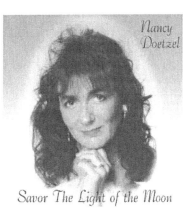

Nancy Doetzel

Savor The Light of the Moon

and Canadian Elvis Tribute Artist Champion.

The concert began with Daylin and I carrying flaming white candles, while walking towards the dim lit stage and singing Joy to the World. After leading a sing along with the audience, we sang two Elvis songs as duets. Then I stood alone, dressed in a white cotton night gown and holding a flaming white candle. Standing beside a young child clad in angel attire, I sang an original song, which I had composed after coming out of surgery, related to cancer, and I called it "Thought about Dancing," As I prayerfully sang this melody, a pin could have been heard dropping, and tears were evident on the faces of those whose hearts were being touched by a message of hope:

There were many angels watching on that frightful August day.
Felt them close beside me, telling me I'd be okay
Lying there while waiting, humming a gospel tune,
Trusting in those angels, in that cold dim room.

I thought about dancing, seeing the bright sunlight
So strong and healthy, I was ready for the fight
Being hit so suddenly by the silent big C
Happens only to others, Is this really me?

Tears rolled down my cheeks, as I counted down,
Prayerfully I fell asleep, dressed in a while gown,
Awakened in an hour, saw the bright sunshine,
Thanked the many angels, toasted with some wine.
I thought about dancing, seeing the bright sunlight,
So strong and so hopeful, I knew I'd won this fight,
Being hit so suddenly with the silent big C,
Not only happens to others, it happened to me..

After a short concert break, Ken and I celebrated our wedding anniversary by waltzing together on stage, while I sang my CD title song, Savour the Light of the Moon:

The blue Danube waltz plays,
she catches his gaze
Flashes the card on her wrist,
He asks her to dance,
Hoping black tails and pants
Would make him hard to resist.

She just wants to keep dancing,
at the Newport Mansion

Waltz gracefully across the room,
savour the light of the moon
Be queen of the ball,
in Beechwood hall
Step into a dream land,
never let go of his hand.

She's Cinderella tonight,
all dressed in white
A long gown and slippers make it right
Couples dance beside her,
they seem like a blur
She's in her own space,
with a smile on her face

The blue Danube waltz ends,
he slowly bends
Bows and kisses her wrist,
Walks on the foyer,
signs her card once more
Escorts her back to the floor.

I felt the joy of altruism during the Christmas season
when I presented the funds raised from the CD launch concert to the Cancer Research Foundation and the Thunder
Bay Regional Hospital Foundation. Before returning to
Calgary, I celebrated the final new years eve of the 20th
century with family in Thunder Bay. In a first new millennium *Thunder Bay Post* newspaper column I wrote:

> The past is history, the future is a mystery and the
> moment is a gift. That is why the moment is called "the
> present." Part of this common belief was reflected last
> Friday night when many people, expressed a strong
> apprehension about the mystery of the future. They
> were fearful of leaving their homes in case the Y2K bug
> somehow kicked in. Fed by the media during the past
> year, this bug became catchy, like a nasty flue epidem-
> ic. Resembling endless static on a radio, it had blocked
> masses from tuning into the merriment of experiencing
> the beginning of a new century. Instead of waltzing
> happily with life, the final moments of the 20th century,

many people had played out the drama of a millennium tragedy, and reacted accordingly.

While shopping in the afternoon, December 31, I noticed people at the checkouts were purchasing candles, flashlights, bottled water and matches. At that point, I started to wonder whether or not I had made the right decision to attend an New Years Eve 2000 celebration at the Royal Canadian Legion, on May Street. Although, I was still set on attending the event, I decided that I should also stalk up on candles, bottled water and matches. Thus it was evident that I had caught the Y2K bug and the stores were going to make a profit on my case.

Before I left my home, to head to a New Years celebration, I checked my house to make sure all my supplies were easily accessible if I needed them. Then, prayerfully, I headed out to the legion in hope of having the opportunity to experience a Y2K bug cure, at midnight The meal was delightful, the band Crystal River was excellent and the celebrants were fun to be with at the legion. When the clock struck midnight, the lights and heat remained on and the band continued to perform. A shared joy with the crowd brought me a heightened state of awareness and a quiet receptivity of the wonderment sensed during such a festive moment. The Y2K bug had been annihilated and a group of celebrants were greeting a new era. This moment truly was a New years present.

I awakened January 1st to the smell of fried eggs and toast. Ken had been cooking a new millennium breakfast which he brought to my bedside on a tray. When he opened the bedroom drapes, I noticed beautiful snowflakes falling from the heavens, like frozen tear drops. I felt my heart aching at the thought of having to leave my treasured husband at home, when I returned to Calgary within a few days. As I savored my breakfast, I could feel my own tear drops falling into my plate. I questioned how I could sacrifice so much to obtain a doctorate. After engaging in a prayer of gratitude, I sensed a sacred voice within my heart, informing me that attending university in Calgary to work towards a doctorate was part of my sacred mission. Then, I recalled a promise to my Creator, en route to surgery after my cancer diagnosis. I had asked for divine healing in return for acceptance of a calling to awaken the inherent latent spirit within anyone the Creator put on my path. I was to become a spiritual doctor to assist others to emerge from caterpillars into butterflies and from acorns to trees.

Before my mother and sister arrived at my home for a traditional seasonal turkey dinner, I visited the Thunder Bay Armoury for a New Years luncheon. I spoke with the mayor and other local politicians who talked about my former community work. They indicated that my newspaper column, radio and television shows and singing performances had given me a strong presence in the city. Again, I found myself feeling a sense of grief for having left Thunder Bay. I attempted to communicate my intentions in a *Thunder Bay Post* column.

> To answer a common question asked by some Thunder Bay Post readers in regards to what drives me to keep on studying and working towards obtaining a doctorate, I will quote Wess Roberts. He states success does not magically arrive as a prize inside a breakfast cereal box. If you want to make something of yourself, no matter what hand you have been dealt, you must have faith in your ability to play your hand in a practical, realistic and sometimes risky way. The quest for success never ends. It must be continued each day. Once a goal has been achieved, it is replaced with another goal related to making the world a better place for everyone.

> Roberts further states that education changes us by releasing us from a prison of ignorance and he says there are no entitlements to personal achievement. You have to make choices as you chart your own destiny each day. On the other hand, he points out, if you're never afraid, you must be crazy. Robert's reflections, on pursuing one's goals despite fear, lead me to recall the first day that I stepped into a PhD class at the University

of Calgary, wondering how my fellow students and professors would view a Lakehead University grad. Could a Thunder Bay girl fit in with some doctorate cow town students and high profile professors, I asked myself. At that time, I felt like I was back in the primary grades again, with fear that I may be rejected by my peers and looked down upon. However, the opposite of what I feared took place. I soon acknowledged that somebody can feel more appreciated in a far away city than in their own home town, where people assume they know him or her well. I soon felt as if obtaining a higher education and being in a larger city were giving me a passport to freedom of expression in the Western World.

Despite what I have just written in this column, I can honestly say there is no place like home, and I am happy to be back in Thunder Bay for a few days. Also I am very grateful to Westject for its direct flight to Calgary and for its staff's first-rate personalities. When I called to inform the staff that my purse was missing, after falling out of my briefcase on a flight, I spoke to some very concerned and understanding employees. Within a few hours, my purse was on a flight back from Hamilton and I was picking it up from the airport. On other occasions, I've noted that some staff had exceeded their job descriptions to help make me feel stress-free on route to Calgary. Also, they have entertained me with their sense of humour and jokes of the day. I hope Thunder Bay does not take these airlines for granted, as we are fortunate to have it in this city, along with staff that appears to love their jobs.

I packed my clothes and books hoping that my suitcases contained everything I needed when I returned to Calgary. Often, after coming home to Thunder Bay, I would need to call Ken and request that he send out some books or clothes that I had left behind. And, it was common for me to have a sense of fragmentation when travelling back and forth between the two cities.

A research methodology class was the first university session that I attended after returning to Calgary, following the Christmas holidays. I had been asked to find examples of qualitative research studies which have different ontological and epistemological understandings of social phenomena and explain and illustrate these differences. I recalled having been taught the standpoint that realism embraces the ontological view that the world has an existence that is independent of our perceptions. People's values determine how human life is structured on the basis of their own reason and purposive action.

As an example of an investigative qualitative research study, I presented a news documentary video, which introduced an alleged "stigmata" case. The production presented from the Fox Studios in Los Angeles was aired on various television stations in November 1999. In the documentary, Katya Rivas, from Bolivia was being observed by a sceptical journalist along with a camera crew, her family and a priest while she had an alleged stigmata experience. The investigative journalist said that he was not relying on his emotionalism to put the stigmata into perspective. But he had concluded that Katya's suffering was no way self inflicted.

This experience of a stigmata was said to have taken place during a Corpus Christie celebration of the Catholic Church's central sacrament of communion, which is the taking of bread and wine as body and blood of Christ. Katya allegedly experienced the "supposed" mental and physical suffering of Christ, during the "estimated" same hours Christ was carrying the cross and being crucified. In the documentary, Katya spoke about Christ using her to communicate to the world about the importance of remembering what His crucifixion stands for. She said Jesus was demonstrating some of his suffering through her stigmata experience. Katya stated that she hoped to connect human hearts with the heart of Christ, which she believed could help transform humanity. She insisted that many people's arrogance keeps them tuned out of their hearts.

After presenting a video clip from this documentary, I spoke to students about how the life of Jesus was recently featured on the television network in a program titled

Biography. The program suggested that Jesus created the greatest social revolution in history; His life changed people's lives and the course of human history. He had a simple message, which is to love one another, but consequently he was put to death on political grounds.

This Biography program indicated that Jesus was illiterate, and before commencing his ministry he had travelled to India to learn some truths from Buddha. During the telecast, the Bible was referred to as being the most powerful popular book in the universe. Apparently, it has been translated into 2000 languages and at least 44 million copies are sold annually. Some scholars have suggested that the Bible has the power to change lives and the whole nation; science may not be able to change human nature, but religious beliefs can. Religion is viewed as a system of thinking that can bring meaning and purpose to life. According to statements made within this Biography program, a current interest in Jesus is big business because of the timeless power of His life and message.

I pointed out to my peers that in the December 1999 issue of *Reader's Digest*, Paul Johnson had written a story indicating that at the threshold of a new millennium, Christianity is alive and well in the minds and hearts of countless believers. He stated that evidence suggests Christianity will still be flourishing another thousand years from now as it continues to strike new roots and regain lost territories. Johnson told readers that it is impossible to travel anywhere in the world, without finding a church, chapel or symbol commemorating Jesus message. Jesus offers a continuing vision of our better, purer selves and the better, purer world we could create. His message is one of tenderness, kindness, compassion, love, faith and hope. Scores of new books are being written by scholars about Jesus and television networks, such as NBC and ABC, are profiling Jesus, as the Miracle worker.

I was confronted by a few fellow students for having addressed Jesus in a university setting. They questioned where He fits into the scholarly world. In a follow-up class presentation, I summarized the context of how Jesus would be written about in my doctorate dissertation, addressing spiritual leadership within education. In my dissertation, I would use some of my reflective journal entries and literature to support a standpoint about the relevance of Jesus as a major mentor of spiritual leadership.

The lives of some great spiritual masters such as Buddha, Muhammad, and Jesus, have provided roadmaps that can assist educational leaders to evolve spiritually. Without a good leader, taking a spiritual path can be like trying to journey in quicksand while ignoring a near-by paved highway, going in the same direction. Although these three leaders all shared a common fate of abandonment and separation from their own communities in their early missions to serve mankind, they each enlightened the world by articulating different aspects of spirituality. Christian teachings suggest Jesus' leadership mission was to give sight to people spiritually blind and demonstrate to individuals who thought they could see that they were blind. Stories about Jesus proclaim that He came into the world as light to awaken the fruits of the spirit: love, joy, peace, patience, kindness, gentleness, fidelity and self control within his followers. Some Christians believe that parables about Jesus' leadership awakened them to their divine nature and that a major change occurred in human nature as a result of the birth, life, death, and ascension of Christ. Followers became more grateful, compassionate, and heart-centred in their treatment of others, which demonstrated they had evolved into becoming more caring individuals.

Like Buddha and Muhammad, Jesus was judged harshly for frequently speaking loudly against injustice, courageously standing up for women's rights and confidently encouraging new ways of thinking. Although Jesus articulated and mentored many divine aspects of leading, spirituality is not restricted to a belief in the Christian God. Buddha, Muhammad and other spiritual leaders who perceived transcendence in non-personal terms also modelled inner peace, social justice and spirituality. Additionally, there are many charitable, caring leaders who do not believe in God, but their active expressions of the divine gives them a sense of joy, wonder, and awe. The holy can appear to us in an encounter with a rock, a bush, a stream, a flower or in the words of Jesus, Buddha and Muhammad.

I have been appreciative of opportunities to incorporate Jesus teachings into my scholarly world, but realize that the true messages of Jesus are ineffable, tacit and visceral. Jesus taught mainly by his mentoring within his actions, which changed people's hearts and demonstrated that actions speak louder than words. He did not write down his messages. Therefore, attempting to articulate understandings of Jesus message is very challenging within an academic setting. Perhaps, this is the reason that the suggestion has been made by some scholars to edit all mention of Jesus out of my doctorate dissertation.

Travelling to and from the university by C-train has given me opportunities to speak openly about Jesus and to do reflective readings and meditation before and after university classes. I am also given chances to meet and converse with interesting people. When on the C-train, one cold winter day, I sat with a young man who claimed he was travelling on the train just to kill time. I asked him why he would want to kill something given to us to be used wisely, not destroyed. Time should never be wasted but used to the best advantage, I told him. Later, I was grateful that he'd chosen to spend some time giving directions on how to get to the church I was heading to. I thought that if a fraction of the time people wasted could be used to make a difference in somebody else's life, or to do something constructive in their own life, the world would become a better place. We can't make up lost time, because it's gone forever.

Two hours of my time that night were consumed listening to Father Hugh Feiss, a Benedictine monk from Oregon, speaking at a church in Calgary. He spoke about the difference between religion and spirituality. His message was that Jesus sought to create an immediate link between God and humankind, not to set up bureaucratic channels to go through. But, he noted that Jesus has been managed, monopolized and codified.

Feiss further suggested that self-righteous fanaticism is associated with being highly religious, rather than spiritual. Spiritual exercises and expressions can be certain physical activities, not just prayers and meditation in churches. Devotion, service and ritual can all be expressions of spirituality. Spirituality inspires a person to give in to an overpowering grace he or she has selected that meets his or her needs. It is searching for and discovering faith in faith.

I recall recently learning about Feng Shui, a spiritual approach to living a balanced life. When I was in Thunder Bay, I had attended the Feng Shui introductory seminar. The speaker, Patrick, had been practising the ancient art of Feng Shui for over twenty-five years. Feng Shui is an ancient Chinese art and science first developed some 6000 years ago. It's a system based on keen observation and experimentation that assumes people are part of a cosmic dance of energy, in flux. Since this energy pervades one's being, if it is not properly harnessed, one's possibilities can be wasted. Feng Shui is the study of environment, places, people, time and how the energies of each interact. It is a practice of understanding and harnessing these forces of energy to benefit one's well being. Placing furniture correctly in one's home is one way of practising Feng Shui. Patrick advised me not to place my bed underneath a window or have it along the same wall as a door opening or between a window with no curtains and a doorway because the free flow of qui gets blocked. He also suggested not living in a house close to many hydro towers, since an electric current could affect the flow of qui.

When talking about the five elements of Feng Shui, which are metal, water, wood, fire and soil, Patrick explained the magic square and how people's dates of birth determine their element. According to my birth date, my element is wood. This means that I would benefit from being in close proximity to trees. For three years in Calgary, I was a tenant at Don's home that had eleven trees on the front lawn and fourteen in the backyard. This location proved ideal for my studying and writing.

One evening when I was reading my reflective notes, I noticed a statement that indicated it is often implied that people holding religious beliefs must be either brainwashed, intellectually challenged or in need of some kind of crutch. I felt like this statement applied to some students' perceptions of my research. I was becoming more aware that society has lost sight of the value of the spiritual part of one's essence.

I appreciated opportunities to share such reflections with a wise elderly friend, Ellafern, who lives in Thunder Bay. After discussing some of my research, Ellafern informed me of her own latest writings. She told me that her love of writing kept her busy working on an autobiography of the first twenty-five years of her life, despite the health challenges she had encountered.

"I feel totally alive when I write," Ellafern said. "I write because the story is there to be told and I have to write it."

Ellafern communicated with me, as if she had known me forever. We were convinced that our personal stories had a spiritual weave that connected us. Whenever, we spoke on the telephone or were together in person, our spirits were uplifted. On St. Patricks Day, I sang "When Irish Eyes Were Smiling" during a visit to Ellafern's home.

I had travelled to Thunder Bay March 17, to sing and dance at a traditional St. Patrick's Day celebration. During the celebration, St. Patrick was honored for his ability to spread faith, love and hope in Ireland. Methodically he was remembered for having chased the snakes out of Ireland so that healthy grapes could continue to be harvested there. Some of my ancestors are of Irish heritage.

When in Thunder Bay to celebrate St. Patricks Day, I heard John Stackhouse, a professor of theology at Regent

College, speak at Lakehead University. In my *Thunder Bay Post* Column, I wrote about his lecture:

> The main focus of John Stackhouse's address was associated with the title of his book, *Can God Be Trusted*. In this book, Stackhouse wrote about the Christian revelation, which promises the transformation of suffering into joy, as the best guide to God's dealings with the world. In his talk he challenged listeners to take responsibility for their actions and to examine the celestial blueprint with less despair. Stackhouse spoke of Jesus as being the human face of God and the Trinity of God in the form of Father, Son and Holy Spirit. He explained that God revealed himself in Jesus, who had life changing powers and represented truth, hope and love. Jesus brought salvation to the world which enables mankind to be reconciled to God.
>
> Scripture is a map on how to live life fruitfully, Stackhouse said. If we want to know what God is truly like, we can look at Jesus, for Jesus mirrors God. Stackhouse explained that although masculine pronouns are used in the scriptures to describe God, traditional theism also affirms that God is not essentially male. God is spirit. Furthermore, God created human beings as male and female, both in God's own image. Thus, it is well for us to keep in mind the feminine aspect of the divine as we consider such a basic question as how God administers the world.
>
> During his address, Stackouse was asked how one should begin believing in God and Jesus. "It's something like taking marriage vows, he said. "You just get into faith and try it." Stackhouse told his audience that God in Jesus declares Godself to us, touches us though the love of others, speaks to us though the Bible and in prayer, and provides for our needs.

After Stackhouse's address, I left the university campus and celebrated St. Urhos day at the Finnish Hall. Methodically, St. Urhos was being honored for having chased the grasshoppers out of Finland to save their crops. The Finnish population established the celebration to coincide with St. Patrick's day. Like the Irish, they dressed in green attire to mark the occasion. With political figures leading the way while carrying a huge plastic grasshopper, celebrants paraded down Bay street, displaying colorful banners that proudly displayed their culture. In my *Thunder Bay Post* column, I described the importance of multicultural events, such as St. Patrick's Day and St. Urhos:

> Many people joining the parade wore a "Multicolored Bow," as a commitment to the "Elimination of Racial Discrimination." The red, yellow, black and white ribbons represented the colours of the human race. They also signified the beauty and harmony created when a diverse people of the world unite together. March 1986, the Prime Minister proclaimed in the House of commons Canada's participation in the Second Decade and said "let us all work toward the day when racism and racial discrimination become history and when every Canadian can participate fully and equally in the life our country." The concept of multiculturalism encompasses all groups in the country. This includes immigrants who have just arrived, those who have been here from generations and the First Nations indigenous people. Every individual and all groups that have become a part of Canada contribute to a multicultural nature. Government policy on multiculturalism is an acknowledgement of a fact of life across the nation as reflected in the population's cultural, racial and linguistic composition.

I celebrated my Irish and Aboriginal heritage when singing and dancing at the Multicultural Association Folklore Festival in Thunder Bay, held annually in the spring. The occasion brought different ethnic, cultural and racial groups together to share their talents and food at the Fort William Gardens. In May, one year, I travelled the Red Eye Air Canada flight from Vancouver to Thunder Bay, so that I could perform at the festival. A late arrival time resulted in me rushing home from the airport, changing into a green gown, grabbing my guitar and speeding over to the festival location. When I was en route, two police officers stopped me and questioned why I was in so much of a hurry. When they noticed my Irish outfit and guitar on the front seat, they smiled and joked that they would escort me to festival. Upon arrival, I could hear my stage call and I started to panic. When the announcer noticed I'd arrived, he made a few jokes with the audience, explaining to them that I had just arrived from Vancouver. When he called me on to the stage, I was out of breath and feared that my hair was probably very messed up. However, I believed the show must go on. Within a few moments, I was belting out the traditional Irish song, "When Irish Eyes are Smiling." When I looked at the audience and noticed that television cameras were filming me, I forgot some of the lyrics, so I hummed until my memory of them returned. It appeared that at least three thousand people were in the audience and I suddenly became aware that television viewers could watch a live telecast of my performance. My stomach was tied in knots and I felt like fleeing the stage. I started to wish that I was back in Calgary, studying alone in my office, far away any public viewing. I sensed that I was exchanging my extroversion for a rebirth of my former introversion.

I had been in Vancouver speaking at a learning love conference, before flying home to Thunder Bay, to perform at the Multicultural festival. In a *Thunder Bay Post* column, I wrote about the Vancouver conference and artist Lila Kane's visit to Thunder Bay the weekend I was on a home visit.

> The love-saturated souls existing within most mothers leads them to express unconditional love towards their children and others. By being loving within their own characters, they can weave care and compassion into the fabric of their own families and communities. That's why May 14 has been marked as a day to honour mothers and cultivate the gratitude they deserve. In the opening ceremonies of a Learning Love Conference held at the University of British Columbia in Vancouver last week, a moment of silence was requested to honour mothers and their roles in mirroring selfless love.

> "Consider our mothers and how they got us here . . . how they helped us to begin our lives," said Sonja

MacPherson, one of the conference organizers. We are not entirely self made. We're made in relationship with others. MacPherson explained that the education system has been guilty of educating children out of the love and compassion their mothers have strived to teach them. Love can be learned and generated through the process of living, she said. We need a more personalized approach to education . . . where love and compassion are central. Some speakers at the conference spoke about how scientific rules and objectivity have hindered love and compassion from developing in students. Cognitive maturity related to an ability to understand and express love is discouraged by a student's fear of being labelled weird or judged as lacking in intelligence. Also, the rugged individualism and a dog-eat-dog attitude promoted in the education system is not student centred and tends to stir up feelings of alienation.

To stress the value of educators mentoring care, one conference speaker quoted Maturana as stating love is that domain of relational behaviours in which another arises as a legitimate other in co-existence with oneself.

Vocalist, chanter, composer, writer and multimedia artist Lila Kane reflects a number of the themes presented at the Vancouver conference. On May 21 at the Unitarian Fellowship, she presented a concert in 7 different languages and 4 varying octaves. "My life is to kiss hearts with song, create a bridge between heaven and earth, share the journey and inspire, for it is not my voice you hear, it is my soul, she said. Voice is the vehicle, music is the gift. May 19 Kane presented a workshop to develop awareness and techniques for mind/body frequencies. She applied the "language of sound while playing rhythm sticks and drums."

During Lila's workshop when participants were chanting, I sensed healing taking place within me. I recall chanting Nam-myoho-Renge-kyo. I had been informed by some physicians that there were suspicions that some of my cells had become abnormal. Within a few weeks, I would be returning to the clinic for a routine check up.

In June, I performed at Benny Birch's Birthday party in Thunder Bay, which was a fundraising event for St. Joseph's Heritage residence for seniors. I had worked at the residence for two years while pursing one of my university degrees and had gained a passion for working with elderly people. I noticed that this population was very childlike and appreciative of people who demonstrated an interest in them. When on stage, I was greeted by a number of the residents who recalled my weekend concerts while working with them. One of my original songs, "Rise up, Let us See," was written to honor this population. Residents had an opportunity to learn the lyrics and sing along, during a celebration held for St. Joseph's Heritage. The lyrics are:

Let us reach our now and show you how
Thankful we are for bringing us so far
The lines on your face are a special grace
Showing wisdom from the years gained from laughter
and tears.

Chorus: Rise up, let us see, how you made history,
You have so much to give and great reason to live
Your love shines through, we believe in you,
Rise up and see, you are free.

You're like children in life's beginning
The light in your eyes, makes you look wise
We want to be there to show we care
You deserve the best, it's time to rest.

As your family, we'd like to be,
There to pray and there to say,
We believe in love and God above
Let's celebrate today, in a special way.

When I was singing this song, one elderly resident stood up in her wheel chair and started to dance. She said she could feel the music in her heart and that it had a healing effect on her. This woman was amongst the crowd who sat close to the stage at Benny Birch's Birthday Party celebration when I was performing.

The way she stood up so tall, and wiggled her toes, reminded me of Tony Melendez playing a guitar with his toes. He was born without any arms. I will go to a Tony Melendez concert when I return to Calgary.

Reflective questions:

What is your meaning of love? How do you express it best towards your self and othrs?

7

Seeking More Truths

I needed to pack my bags to return to Calgary to school after having spent several months in Thunder Bay. I felt torn within heart again, as if I was uprooting myself from a strong foundational lifestyle in a familiar city. I now was going to return to a large unfamiliar city and live in a residence there. Somehow, this all sounded too foreign to me. However, I was very excited to be taking two summer courses that addressed "spirituality." Tad was one of my professors. In my first class with him, he announced to his students that he was dying of cancer and we would be the last group to be taught by him. I could not withhold my tears when I listened to him share his story. For the main course assignment, he asked the students to keep a journal and hand it in at the end of the two week course. He suggested students commence journal entries with a credo. From my heart, I expressed my intentions, by writing:

My Creed is to reflect the sacred, spiritual elements of leadership by caring and nurturing my own soul and the souls of others. I will savour simplicities-love that is true, wonder that is childlike, and humility that is home grown. While reaching out to others through love, compassion and forgiveness, I will revel in the chance to be helpbul to another soul in need. However, I will try to act without expecting to receive any recognition or reward. Time will be set aside daily for me to observe my surroundings until I find evidence of the sacred and view it as a miracle. I will study a sacred text to find a concept that stirs my soul. Before going to sleep, I will review my actions during the day, count my blessings and pray for someone in need. Each night when I retire, I will pray that I have made at least one human being a little happier, or a little wiser or at least a little more content with himself or herself. I can always light up the lamp of faith in my heart with a prayer which will lead me safely through the mists of doubt. I will strive to inspire love, hope and courage in leadership, by being a strong role model and giving advice by example. I believe the world does not require so much to be informed as reminded. Thus, instead of criticizing others and finding fault with the actions of others, I will examine myself and correct my own faults.

I refuse to be a dancer who blames the drummer for my wrong steps. Building a better me is what I will strive to accomplish daily. While self-evolving, I will aim to reflect love itself and love's family of enabling, ennobling and expanding virtues. I will pray for the courage not to be thwarted by fear, as courage makes love possible. I will strive to keep my love fluid, so it can fill whatever vessel life places before me. As an angel with only one wing, I can fly only by embracing another with love, hope and courage. I will greet each day with love in my heart. Love is all that people have not sufficient imagination to exaggerate the importance of. I believe hate is a toxin that poisons the well springs of the soul.

I will love in a way that when I die, my death notice won't appear on a list of life improvements. To make a difference in the world, I will continuously work on developing a better me. I will bathe in the golden glow of enthusiasm and seek the seed of triumph in every adversity. My courage and faith will not allow me to be destroyed by adversity. All things shall pass. A gem cannot be polished without friction and I can't work towards becoming my full potential self without facing trials. When my heart cries for what it has lost, my spirit will laugh for what it has found. I will aim to work like I don't need the money, love like I've never been hurt and dance like nobody is watching. I will learn as if I will live forever and live as if I will die tomorrow. I will apply Dr. Vernon Woolf's tracking methods to potentialize healthy holodynes.

TO KEEP HEALTHY, I will aim to:

a. Retain peace of mind. This involves keeping my thoughts pure through engaging in prayer and meditation.
b. Live in the moment. I must not crucify myself between the two thieves: regret of yesterday and fear of tomorrow.
c. Always affirm inwardly. I am ageless. I am eternal. I live in timelessness. I was created before the galaxies were formed.
d. Acknowledge my life is worth living, so that my belief will create the fact.
e. Note that illness is not something a person has. It's another way of being.
f. Become enthused, no matter what I am doing.
g. Thank God for my health daily and savour life one day at a time.

Throughout my journal entries, which were handed into Tad for marking, I express ways that I am applying his teachings to my life. I wrote:

This course is altering my perceptions of truth in a number of ways. It is giving me new lenses to examine my beliefs through. I am becoming aware that my understanding of spirituality has been bleached of certain perceptions. However, when I am experiencing spirit, all the fragments of my being appear to carry a moment of truth in them.

I learned from Tad that when people experience traumas, lesions in consciousness tend to distort their future development; a false self system begins to grow over their actual self that is repressed. Such traumas can result in aspects of one's awareness being split off into separate little selves that remain at the level of development they had when they were split off. The fragments hide in a part of self which is guarded by a lie. Consequently, a person may be deterred from reaching his or her full potential.

Comparable to Tad's viewpoint about the effects of trauma, I felt aspects of my awareness being split off from my being, when I was informed that my brother had been murdered; and, I have sensed having bruises in my psyche, inflicted by certain injustices in life. However, Shamans have assisted me to heal from some traumas by helping me to recover parts of my being that had become dissociated.. I am valuing many experiences in this class where we are studying Wilber's writing and learning ways our professor is attempting to battle his cancer, by embracing a strong sense of purpose. Some of his classes are stirring up my emotions. Hearing about my professor having been diagnosed with cancer and only given a certain period of time to live, brings me back to the moment I was informed of my own cancer diagnosis. When I think back, I feel very grateful that I am still alive and I am in a class that I love. This professor is more excellent than excellent and so is his class. I do not want to be anywhere else but here, right now, gaining wisdom from his teachings. I am appreciating living my passion of continuous learning.

During a class discussion, we are suggesting that "spiritual democracy" is respecting other's values and beliefs. We agree with Tad that religion, like science is a tool that can be used to transform hatred to love or alternatively do the opposite. However, the simple expression of a caring heart can equal religion, and love and compassion do reflect a universal religion. People have claimed sacredness in their religion and then wiped out a whole species. Such destructive action is definitely not communicating love and compassion.

After attending Tad's classes, it seems like I am examining church through a different lens and paying closer attention to the messages within a sermon. One Sunday morning, the pastor spoke about whimpering spirits, needing to be fed by God, and about some people searching for something to fulfil their taste buds, like a person craving sweets, and then seeking out chocolate pie. The searchers do know what chocolate pie tastes like, so they search different churches and places to find what their taste buds are looking for. When they recognize the correct ingredients and recipe in a certain location, they say "yummy" and then beg for more.

In his sermon, this same pastor suggested that Jesus can be an irritant to the world, like an oyster is an irritant to the shell that provides a pearl.Divine love can irritate some people, like pouring hot coals on a person's head. Jesus' love and compassion and caring did irritate some observers of his actions, who doubted His sincerity.

At the end of semester we hand in our journal entries to Tad for him to review. After his final class, we compose and sing a farewell song to him:

Tad is our teacher, we all see
Teaching us all to be
More spiritual in our own way,
To Live just for today.
Tad's helped us to understand,
That a woman and a man,
Are equal in God's eyes,
Are meant to have sacred ties.

He's taught us lot about love,
To see God, below and above,
To search for truth each day,
And respect what others say.

After standing beside Tad, and singing for him, we all embrace him and express how thankful we feel for being students in his final class. I feel like I do not ever want his course to end, but I know the topic will continue to be part of my life learning.

Tad died on June 24, 2001. He was diagnosed with cancer several years before he died, but minor surgery appeared quite successful. Then, Tad experienced a recurrence in 2000, and was told that he had one to two years to live. A few excerpts from the e-mail Ken Wilber sent to Tad and his wife Noreen on April 17, 2000 were shared with some of his students:

I am deeply saddened by the news . . . one to two years they have given you. Still (and I have this on rather good authority), one to two years can be an eternity. I certainly do not mean to make light of the situation, it is just that the last few years that Treya and I had seemed like decades, because time expands in proportion to how much it is valued. I valued every second, every second contained years. Of course I wish the years could be just the good old chronological years – another 30 for each of us, say – but in lieu of that, there is at least the possibility that two years lived with thankfulness for each moment are qualitatively a lifetime of years lived unaware.

Wilber's statement about time "lived with thankfulness for each moment are qualitatively a lifetime of years lived unaware" seemed like a tattoo of sacred words engraved on my heart. When the doctor had suggested that I may live for six months, I told my husband that I had already sensed that I had lived a hundred years up until my diagnosis. I knew that I had been living life to the fullest, with great passion, while appreciating the rewards of choices I had made. Every moment can be a blessing, if we look for ways to be grateful. Having lost my father and brother when they were both very young led me to realize that none of us are promised tomorrow. But, I also know and accept that we are all given free will and we do reap the benefits and consequences of our choices.

I am being reflective of Tad's argument that the truth will indeed set us free, but only if we recognize that there is more than one truth. I acknowledge that I have been socialized to see life in a certain way, which could be much different than how my friends view their own lives. Letting go of absolutes and perceiving my truth as just being a partial truth is challenging, but this view point does reflect my sociological teachings. I am aware right now that what is . . . just is, and I am thankful to be taking a break from school to travel.

Reflective question: What is your mission and your credo?

8

Reverence of Divine Grace

It's time to return to Thunder Bay, before taking a major trip with Ken to Rome. I am very excited when I hop on a Westjet flight, heading home to meet Ken and prepare for another pilgrimage. I am just in Thunder Bay one day, before boarding a flight to travel to Rome. I question whether or not my lost dairy will show up in one of the airports we stop at. I am still wondering if it is in someone's hands, or part of the soil at a garbage dump.

While not being able to sleep, when on the long flight to Rome, I am thinking of situations when I needed to talk things through and nobody was there; times when I chose the wrong person at the wrong time to share laughter or pain; times when I needed to just cry to make my sorrow conscious and to bring closure to an experience so I could move on. I am aware that my personal growth is not linear. After many peak experiences, I've moved forward and upward, but then have sensed going downward and backward when encountering challenges. Now, I am questioning if the pilgrimage in Rome will have a further healing effect me. I am intending on meeting the Pope for the second time.

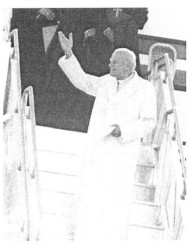

The first time I met Pope John Paul was when I was in the role of a journalist, covering the story of his visit to Winnipeg. I was with a group of other reporters from around the world, at the Winnipeg airport when he arrived. I was teased by the other journalists for acting so excited about the event. Despite all the security surrounding him, when he arrived, he reached out his hand, blessed my forehead, and called me an angel. I truly felt blessed and privileged. However, the privilege of receiving communion from him was taken away from me when the RCMP escorted me down a platform leading to where he was giving out communion at Bird's Hill Park. They stated that I was wearing a journalist accreditation tag, not the tag of a Nun or Priest.

Ken and I are with the group at the Vatican. Again, I am feeling elated to be here. I am dressed in a white outfit and sitting behind a group of Nuns, also wearing white clothing. When a call goes out over the sound system requesting those who require healing, to head towards the front stage, I follow the Sisters up to the platform where Pope John Paul is sitting, and I receive another healing blessing from Him. When our Pilgrimage leader notices my absence from the group, he informs Ken that I may have to spend a night in jail for having presented myself as a counterfeit Sister at the Vatican. However, after I receive the Pope's blessing, I joyfully return to my seat and join the group. They notice I appear very healthy and energetic.

We are walking down the cobalt streets, touring many incredible Cathedrals and Churches. I am feeling the uplifting divine effects of continuous prayer, despite my jet lag. I wear out the soles of my shoes when walking the streets, so Ken and I wonder away from the pilgrimage group to find me some new shoes. The shoes in the stores are very high fashion but not comfortable to wear. I walk on bare feet until we find a jean pair of sandals. Then we purchase some wine and sit on a wall overlooking Rome, while I compose a new song and dance up and down a stairway that appears to be heading towards heaven. I am celebrating being in a very beautiful sacred place, far away from my scholarly world.

Before returning to Calgary, Ken and I spend two days in Venice. We travel by a Gondola on the canal to arrive at our hotel. The pouring rain never ceases while we are there, and touring the area is like being in a labyrinth. We are strangers to the land, and often lost. Beneath the cloudy skies, many of the buildings appear to be duplicates in design. However, I sense mystery and romance as we trek throughout the village, holding hands. I am wondering where the moon and stars are hiding. I am wishing I could sing and dance in the rain. I love the music and rhythm of the thunder.

It is time for us to return to Thunder Bay and then I will go back to Calgary to attend my university classes. I am finding it difficult to return to school and continue my research. Westject enables me to work at the *Thunder Bay Post* as a reporter in Thunder Bay on a Monday morning, and still arrive at the University of Calgary, to go to my research class the same day. The flight is just over two hours. When I arrive, I speak to fellow students about how I had conducted observational research, while on my pilgrimage. I have definitely become more awakened spiritually while on this venture, and returning to an educational institution is somewhat challenging.

It is a few days, after returning to Calgary from the pilgrimage. I've have had a long day at school and my brain feels over loaded. I need to do something physical to get out of the cerebral mode. I go to a church to take a dance class, after working out in the gym close by. There are not enough males to accommodate all the female students. I am dancing alone beside a pole, feeling like an ugly girl at a prom. After I put my running shoes on to leave, another dance student, Mohamed arrives and asks if I need a partner. I am not sure why, but I sense that I know him from some where else. We dance a waltz and cha cha together. In the following weeks, he returns to the other dance classes, so that I will have a partner. After taking lessons together, we commence a sacred friendship.

During Ramadan, Mohamed shares readings from the Koran, and I share readings from the Bible. For one week, I fast with him from dawn until sunset. We have an appreciation and respect for one another's religious beliefs, and acknowledge commonalities in our faith. When reviewing the Koran and Bible together, we note both Holy Books convey strong messages about needing to keep our hearts pure, and being caring and compassionate people, who serve God, who created us. We both are aware that most Christians are not encouraged to read the Koran, and the majority of Muslims choose not to read the Bible. However, Mohamed reminds me that Muslims do speak freely about how their Holy Book acknowledges that Jesus was implanted in the womb of a young woman named Mary. The Koran indicated that Jesus was "a word" of God and a special sign for humanity. He was the result of a miracle, and consequently, miraculous things began to take place.

I truly appreciate opportunities to share commonalities and differences in Mohamed and my belief systems, during our breaks at dance classes. I feel like my spirit is being uplifted by our discussions, dances and prayers. I also enjoy all the laughter we share when I step on his toes, while trying to learn new dance steps. The scuffs on his shoes show evidence of me having two right feet. But, I thank God that I have feet, even if they don't always do what I want them to do.

At a seasonal dance, on the university campus, I meet a group of other students taking time out from their studies. I am grateful for a chance to be together with others who have a passion for dancing. A group of us sit on the university campus steps and share humorous stories about our lives. When we are laughing and continuing to dance outdoors, it appears like we are intoxicated from drinking alcohol. But, our true beverage of choice is Diet Pepsi. While having so much fun, I am hoping not to be noticed by some serious scholars, walking by carrying their books, en route to study. I am feeling a bit guilty for not being at my desk, beside my computer, typing.

I am grateful when I have time out from my university classes. The sun is shining very bright and it is an ideal day to spend in Banff. I want to go hiking in the mountains. I sense that I require some physical, mental and spiritual healing. I am encountering pain in my spinal cord, and finding it difficult to walk. Neil drives me to go hiking and climbing at a refreshing mountain location in Banff. I am struggling in the climb, but feel the mountains hugging my whole being as we ascend in our climb. There are lakes and waterfalls soothing my soul, as I rest from the climb. Some snow is capping the mountains. I fall a few times, as we are descending.

Towards the end of the descent, I notice a huge grizzly bear and want to go pet it, as if it was a friendly puppy. I recall an Aboriginal Elder telling me that I was from the bear clan, and that a bear would never harm me. I have memories of my mother speaking about a bear sniffing my toes when I was a baby resting in a play pen. I walk towards the bear, fearlessly, as Neil video tapes me. I speak to the bear, as if it is human and request that it take away my pain from my spinal chord and send me healing energy. When my eyes caught him looking upwards, I sensed that we had established some kind of heart to heart connection. I felt my pain subside and my spirit uplift. Other hikers stood very still on the path, appearing frozen on the spot, probably questioning whether or not I was suicidal, or crazy.

I return to my residence feeling very uplifted and peaceful. The physical discomfort has lightened. When I arrive, I am informed that there is mail for me, delivered personally by the landlord, Don. I have just received a letter from a university in Beijing, asking me to speak about "spiritual intelligence" at an upcoming conference in China. I feel very honored, and apply for funding the next day. Then, within a few months, I am en route to China, questioning how this could ever have happened. When I arrive at the airport, fear strikes me and I feel paralyzed. I am not sure the name of my hotel, or where the conference is taking place, because I accidentally left my file with this information on, in the airport. A Chinese woman, who was sitting beside me on the plane, assists me in locating which hotel that I am supposed to go to. The Taxi driver she flags down for me does not speak English and he drops me off at a hotel with "no name." I feel like screaming, but suddenly I spot my friends Stephanie and Richard, who are from China, but work at the University of Calgary. Their hugs are like a breath of fresh air that makes me feel grateful for this opportunity to travel to China.

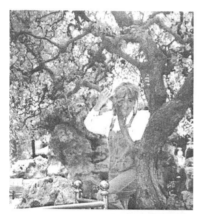
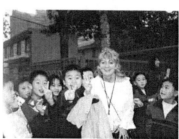
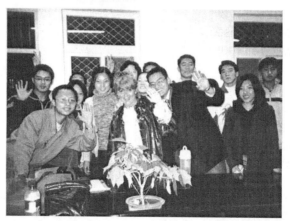

In Beijing, I am climbing the Great Wall and feeling in awe, while writing in my diary. I have braids in my hair and I am wearing jean coveralls. It appears very strange to me, that tourists are photographing me when I look like I am ready to go fishing. I definitely do not appear like a scholar, reflecting on a presentation to be given the following day at the university. The scenery from the Great Wall is incredible and I feel like I have just stepped into a postcard. The climb upwards is breathtaking and very meditative. I have an incredible sense of peace. I am in awe and feel like staying there, and observing the sun setting.

I have just spoken to a university class at the University of Beijing. I talked about heart wisdom and shared my story of surviving cancer, to date. One student in the classroom, Richard, appeared very familiar to me, when he entered the class room where I was speaking. After I finished speaking, he asked if I would sing "My Heart Goes On" for the students. When I sang this song, all the students sang along with me. I was amazed that they knew this song so well. Richard later insisted that I had an old heart. He said that he believed in reincarnation and that he must had known me in another life. His assumption appeared to merit some possibility, when we exchanged stories of common dreams and memories. For several hours, while touring the Forbidden City, we spoke about our lives, as if we were siblings. When he bid farewell, he said he felt as if his heart had been cleansed. He claimed he felt like he wanted to work towards making a major difference in the world.

After I arrive home from China, I notice that Ken is not well. He appears to be over stressed from being a vice president of a company for so many years and because I am away from home now. While working on my doctorate, I have not been spending time going out dancing or attending major entertainment acts at the Community Auditorium like we had done frequently in the past to relax. I am residing in Calgary now, and attending university. My doctorate research appears to have become like a "second spouse." I am sleeping with books at night and appearing to be hugging computers, while typing continuously on word. I am living and breathing my research. I am missing taking walks to the shores of Lake Superior with Ken. I am longing for my former lifestyle. I am living a very lonely life, while studying.

Ken's life style has also become off balance and he is displaying symptoms of being a workaholic. He is expressing that he is unsure about how he would like to spend his future. He is talking about becoming single again, getting a motor bike and travelling across the country alone. I am trying not to react emotionally to his voiced intention. But, I can feel my heart ripping, as he shares what he would like to do. Although I am certain that my divine calling and mission is to finish my doctorate, I am also sure that my marriage to Ken is sacred and valued. I intend to honor my commitment made to him at the church alter more than once. I promised to take him . . . for better . . . and for worse . . . in sickness and in health. Therefore, I feel like forgetting about finishing my doctorate, and alternatively joining him on a bike ride across the country.

I reflect on an occasion when Ken and I had talked about taking a bike ride across Canada. We were attending a retreat called, The Wall, held in the mountains close to Vancouver. At this event, we examined the walls that were preventing us from reaching our full potential selves. And, we were being given suggestions on how to rise above these walls. When reading my journal writings, from this retreat, I find a page where I have written some reflections:

Nobody is really aware of bits of my spirit that are hidden within my songs and journal entries. I feel re-inspired and re-spirited when I read them. I have always loved to commune with nature and find myself in the divine surroundings within a forest. I aim to be like a river always pushing forward, never backwards, whispering, not yelling; reflecting light; existing in the moment; accepting rain and sunshine, mirroring peace, despite barriers encountered in the process of self transcendence; moving towards something larger; like a rock that is strong, unique, colorful, sparkling, looking polished; comparable to a tree that is grounded by its roots and nurtured with branches reaching out to the heavens; resembling a flower that is colorful, smiling, perennial and blossoming.

I recall having used music to communicate some of my deepest feelings to Ken throughout our marriage. Sometimes when he came home from work, and I wanted to tell him that I was upset or happy, I would express my feelings in a song. Thus, I am inspired to write him a song called "With Tears there's a Rainbow."

In one of the verses, I sang:

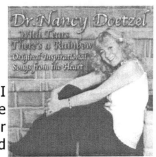

The blessings that we shared,
And all the times that we dared,
To repeat our vows again,
Meant our love would never end.

I send Ken a copy of the song, I have written. I remind him of the many times we have renewed our vows. I apologize for living and breathing my research. But, I do not hear from him for a while. He is supposedly travelling in the Toronto area. I am encountering some kind of illness that makes me suspicious that cancer has returned to my body. I go to the hospital because I am experiencing a lot of pain and I am throwing up blood. I am wondering if my illness is a manifestation of feeling somewhat heart broken. When I am at the hospital, a doctor attempts to contact Ken, but is unable to reach him. A student has taken me to the hospital. I am feeling very weak and in pain.

After I return to my place of residence, Don takes me for a drive to Banff where I can experience a healing hug from the mountains. I am very deficient in energy. I find it difficult to stop crying. My inner tears are being expressed in how I breathe and speak. I am feeling as if knives are being driven through my stomach. I cannot eat. I savor the beauty of the mountains, which remind me that I can rise above my circumstances. I am determined to keep keeping on. Don tells me that I am his angel, who helped him to quit drinking and stop taking drugs. He asks me what he can do to help me get well. He holds my hand and prays for God to heal his angel.

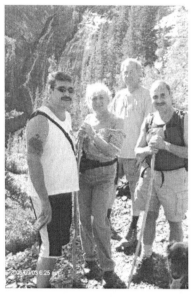

I seek advice from a medical doctor the next day. I am informed that it appears like I have a few tumors that may require surgery. I am aiming to heal from whatever is taking place within my body. Don, Mohamed and Neil assist me in dealing with my health circumstances. They rotate in taking me to the clinic and helping me retain a healthy mindset. Good friends, laughter, dancing, singing and communing with nature are some of my best medicine. I am determined to get well.

I am scheduled to speak at an International conference in Waikiki very soon. My bags are partially packed and I am almost ready to go. Ken will accompany me on the trip. My topics are "Leading from heart and mind" and "Appreciative Inquiry." I will be speaking about the importance of seeing a glass half full, instead of half empty.

An appreciative inquiry process can cultivate heart wisdom. It has been used to enrich spiritual development, heal people's wounds, and enhance personal relationships. Our choices of words within conversations assist in the creation of our reality. Therefore, we should speak of delight, not dissatisfaction; speak of hope, not despair. We should let our words bind up wounds, not cause them to others. Our words can be like healing medicine or poisonous. What we believe to be true is true in its consequences. Our realities are usually based on ten percent of what happens to us and ninety percent of how we choose to perceive our experiences. Being given free will means we can choose how to view and react to whatever happens to us. Looking at a glass with half the water missing, leaves us with a choice to see it as being half full.

I arrive in Hawaii during rainy season and wear my boots to the beach. After reviewing my presentation on the plane, about appreciative inquiry, I am aiming to practice what I am about to preach. I see the beauty in the rain. But, I also celebrate when the sun starts to shine while I am doing a presentation in a room overlooking the ocean. I hear music in the room next door. I later discover it is Paul Pearsal, the author of the book, *The Hearts Code*. Coincidently, I had been speaking about his book in my presentation. He happens to be speaking at another event next door to the Educational conference I am attending. We meet and exchange stories about our research, related to heart intelligence. I inform him about my radio show called "From the heart." He says I have an old heart, but a youthful spirit.

Paul Pearsal speaks to me about heart transplant patients taking on the memories of their donors. He also shares his story of being a cancer survivor. In his presentation, he says that our hearts do not exclusively love and feel; our hearts also think, remember and communicate with other hearts; 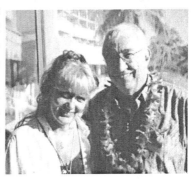 they are the essence of who we are.

Paul suggests to me that an ideal time to receive healing from the ocean is when the sun is setting. It is during sunset. I have decided to take a stroll along the peaceful ocean shores. The waves are rushing in, creating a soothing ambiance. I am feeling a sense of balance with the light meeting darkness. I am sensing that I have just stepped into a beautiful photo of an incredible sunset. I kick off my shoes and walk towards to on-coming waves. Suddenly, the tide comes in and I am pulled into an irresistible current. I am bobbing up and down as the waves and current thrust me far away from the shore. I start to panic and scream, but it appears like nobody is watching or listening. I am under water gasping for air. I am reliving memories of when I had pneumonia and required an oxygen tent to breathe. I sense that I may be losing consciousness. In my mind, I can see and hear my friends saying "we are awaiting your return." I start to pray, like my father had taught me to do. Within a short time, two incredible swimmers are embracing me and carrying me to shore, as they hold hands and swim against the strong current. My tears are adding more salty water to the ocean, as I weep continuously. Again, I ask: can this really be happening to me? Am I in the midst of another miracle unravelling?

Ken and I stay away from the ocean during sunset, after this scare. We take walks in mid afternoon. I seem to be experiencing some kind of post trauma after the event. When I spoke to some known Hawaiian healers at the conference, they explained that the current during sunset may have been strong enough to transmit energy through my body that could have shrunk my tumors. They insisted I probably had received some healing when I was under water, thinking that I may be drowning.

We return to Calgary after a two week getaway. I am sad to bid Ken farewell, as he heads back to Thunder Bay. I start questioning my mission again, wondering if getting a doctorate is the right thing to do. I am feeling homesick for Thunder Bay and my old life style, filled with lots of entertainment and dancing with Ken. I sense very strongly when I am in Hawaii that Ken is struggling with my absence and his responsibilities as vice president of a company.

I am back in university classes, showing off my tan to fellow students and sharing stories about the conference. I am thrilled to have met scholars from all over the world who demonstrated an interest in my research. I am feeling a strong shove in the direction of completing my university work and moving on.

I am en route to the university on a foggy day, when my cell phone rings. I am shocked to hear the words "I love you" before I even said hello. I hear Ken's voice, on the receiver, and it has a different tone than in previous calls. He is now informing me that he has changed his mind about travelling across the country on a motor bike. He says whatever he was experiencing is his own "stuff." He says that when he was in Toronto, he had a dream that I had died of cancer, and that he had gone up to the stage during a graduation celebration, to receive my doctorate, on my behalf. He spoke about waking up, feeling as if the dream was real. He asks me what gift he can give me for my up-coming birthday.

It's a special birthday and I am expecting Ken to fly to Calgary to share the occasion with me. I rush home from school, believing he will be at Don's awaiting my arrival and having a bouquet of flowers. Ken is always known for bringing me flowers and surprising me on my birthdays. My friends are waiting for me at a hall, where a cancer research fundraising event is taking place, as a celebration of my birthday. People had purchased tickets for the occasion and some of the celebrants had volunteered to have their heads shaved to raise additional funds. While waiting for Ken, I am late for the event. When I arrive, my friends are waiting for me with cake and gifts and a readiness to party. Don, Mohamed and Neil have all invited guests from their friendship circles. I sing a joyful song, but I feel very sad while trying to belt out the lyrics to a song I usually sang for Ken... I want him to be present so he I can share my gratitude for being alive, after having been told I may not live to see this Birthday.

I try to smile, as I observe friends having their heads shaved to raise funds. I do my best to dance with the group, but I feel so sad and so alone. A few times, I go outdoors and let my tears blend with the pure white snow flakes that are falling from the heavens. I take a short walk, and observe my footprints behind me, on a snowy trail where puddles of tears follow me. I stick out my tongue and allow the snow to give me a fresh taste, as I picture myself sticking my tongue out at Ken for not attending my party. Then, I laugh at myself and head back into the hall, ready to dance and have fun. It is time to let go of any hurt feelings and live in the joy of the moment.

Ken sent money for me to go buy flowers. I purchase roses and put them beside my computer, so I can savor them while I work on my research, after the celebration. He apologizes for not attending the party and explains that he was away on business. He promises that he and I could celebrate a belated birthday somewhere else soon. When I tell him I am heading to Halifax to speak at a conference, he says he will meet me there.

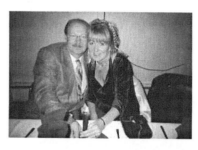

I am staying in a women's dorm in Halifax when Ken arrives, carrying a suitcase and a specially wrapped gift. I need to let him enter through a back door, and sneak him into my dorm. I only have a tiny room and a single bed. Ken thinks this is okay. He hands me a photograph of him and I sitting beside a waterfall at sunset in Thunder Bay. We both look very content and peaceful. There is a symbolism of the sun setting on our past, inviting a new beginning in our relationship.

Ken attends my presentation at the conference. I speak about heart wisdom and spiritual intelligence. Seeing him in the audience is a new and unique experience. He appears surprised as he learns more about the research that I have been conducting about heart and mind synergy, while being a doctorate student in Calgary. After the presentation, he asks me out on a date.

We go for dinner close to Peggy's Cove. Watching the waves wash upon the shores is very soothing and a reminder to live in the now. After communing with nature en route, back to the university dorms, we rent a cabin where we spend the evening nestled within the forest. I feel as if I am back in high school, and first meeting Ken. Ken and I had met when I was seventeen, and in my final year of high school. Now, here we are years later, when I am in my final year of university . . . again, laughing, chatting and dancing in the moonlight outside of a log cabin. We need to leave early the next morning so I can return to the university and Ken can catch his plane back to Thunder Bay. We set out at sunrise, reflecting on a new beginning. Ken promises me that he will move to Calgary soon, and we will renew our marriage vows again.

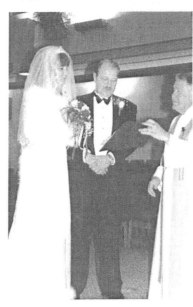

I sit beside the harbor and start composing another song, after Ken leaves. Then I return to the university and meet with other scholars, and I take my flight back to Calgary. The flight appears very long, but I am able to complete some assigned readings.

I read a book. I have promised to write a review about. It is written by a woman, who shares a common tragedy with me. I find it both painful and joyful to read knowing that she and I both experienced the loss of our brothers, in a violent way. I write the following book review for the Catholic magazine, *The Carillon*.

Annette Standwick, author of the book: "Forgiveness: The Mystery and Miracle: Finding Freedom and Peace at last," tugged at my heart strings when she shared her story of being released from the anger and pain of her brother's tragic murder. After having had a common experience of working towards healing from the excruciating pain of knowing that my brother was also murdered, her story enabled me to revisit the mystery and miracle of forgiveness. Even though tears and emotions erupted as I read her book, her story gave me an opportunity to give voice to my grief, and to appreciate the divine power of forgiveness.

Anette writes that people "hurt one another knowingly and unknowingly; intentionally and unintentionally; people have hurt each other from the beginning of time." And the list of losses people experience in a lifetime, that trigger anger and fear are unlimited, she says. The grieving process for hurts and losses includes "denial, anger, bargaining, depression, acceptance and hope." One major way of bringing hope to the hurting person is to bring God into the picture as a partner and then to introduce prayer as an action. God understands pain and loss, for "He too lost his only son, Jesus, to the hands of murderers who beat him and nailed him to the cross."

Healing needs to be experiential to be effective, Annette says. After a person grieves his or her losses, a sense of compassion for the one who caused the hurt may develop. "While compassion does not justify their actions, it can be very helpful when you begin to understand that the hurtful one may be stuck in their own woundedness." Individuals who sense compassion for the one who caused them hurt are able to commence letting go of the wound, enabling them to move towards forgiveness.

Annette points out that "when people find a way to forgive, they become more open to receiving joy, love and satisfaction in their life." She indicates that the healing process involves finding a means to serve others, in spite of the wound. Writing her book enabled her to become transformed by forgiveness. In her book, she states: "I will let you glimpse how God used the aftermath of a human atrocity to transform my undeserving heart, setting me in a direction, I would never have chosen on my own."

Anette, Margot and I shared a table together at a self - publishing meeting, one Saturday morning. We were given a chance to talk about our intentions for books. On the plane, I had an opportunity to review notes that I had written when at the meeting. Margot openly revealed stories about regularly seeing spirits, having visions and roaming outside of her body. She has now written a book about her experiences called *The Exquisiteness of Being Human.*

Reflective questions:

Is there anybody in your life who you need to forgive for the sake of your own wellbeing?

Can you forgive youself for mistakes you've made knowing that to error, is to be human?

9

Moving On

Margot reviewed a draft of my dissertation, when I was in Halifax. She notes that my draft is missing a subjective component and she suggests moving some main points in the ending chapters up to the beginning of the document. Her feedback is very helpful and it assists me in getting on track with my writing. She appears to truly understand what I am aiming to communicate on a topic very challenging to articulate.

While working on making changes to my dissertation draft, I am noticing how stressful I am becoming. One afternoon, I walk to Midlake to rest on a bench and meditate, beside the water. Within a few minutes, I fall into a deep sleep. Something suddenly awakens me, and when I open my eyes, I am surrounded by five beautiful deer. They appear to be watching over me like guardian angels. I sense their presence is some kind of divine message for me reminding me . . . to keep the the faith that I will finish my dissertation.

I return home and start to edit my document. Out of the window in my office, I observe a colorful sunset and hours later, a beautiful sun rise, as I work on completing the final draft of my dissertation. I have a deadline to meet. A cedar candle is burning in my office and relaxing classical music is playing in the background. I am sensing that I will be giving birth to a new document shortly after the sun rises. My labor pains are starting to cease, as I watch my printer transfer the document from the computer screen into print. I have some data typed within heart diagrams and I can see them clearly on the sheets of paper, piling up beneath the printer. I want to yell and scream to express the joy and gratitude that I am feeling.

It is 8 a.m. the morning of the day that I have been requested to hand my completed document. I take a walk, meditate and prepare to bring my sacred document to Office Depot to have copies made for all my doctorate committee members. I carefully pick the document up off the printer, as if it is a child, and then I cautiously wrap it for protection. I leave the house, enter my car and turn on the stereo. The song: "You lift me up" is playing on the radio. My heart beat seems to synchronize with the drum beat in the song.

Several weeks after handing over the copies of my dissertation to my committee members, I am preparing for my defense of my research. I practice defending it almost every evening before sunset. I go to a photographer to have graduation photos taken, in anticipation of graduating in the fall. Then, the day of the exam finally arrives.

Ken drives me to the university. When I arrive, I enter into the examining room and observe my committee members waiting to question me about my research, during a two hour time slot. I look around the room, and notice a painting of a Saint on the wall. Whenever, my mind goes blank, I look at the picture and then feel more relaxed. The questions asked are very tough, but I know that I have spent countless hours preparing for this day. I will just do my best to reflect on the literature and my research findings to answer each question. I am sensing being an anachronism with a very old heart. I am aware this is an anniversary on when I was told I may only live for six months.

After two hours, I am asked to leave the room while the committee makes its decision whether or not I pass the exam. Ken is waiting in the main office, when I exit the examining room. I feel like I am sitting on needles and pins as I await the committee's decision. Then, suddenly there is a bell ringing in the main office, and I am being congratulated for having passed the exam. The committee then addresses me as Dr. Doetzel, for the first time, but I am too numb to respond.

Now, I am wondering what life will be like within my new role as a doctor, rather than a student. I question whether or not I should change my fashions in clothing and hair styles, to better fit my new role. I ponder on where to look for employment opportunities. I start to feel like I am experiencing some kind of grief. I ask myself how I could invest so much time and energy into something that suddenly ends so quickly.

I am preparing for my graduation. My family has traveled from Thunder Bay to share the experience. I am dressed in a long black skirt, with a black vest, white blouse and black tie. I am feeling very nervous as we drive to the university. I 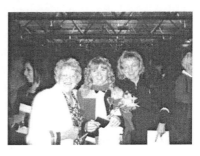 enter the campus and search for the location to dress in my graduation gown. I am asked to sign a sheet to receive my gown and a document. The professor requesting signatures, asks if I am old enough to be a doctor. I am finding it very difficult to believe that I will be walking up on a stage to receive my doctorate degree. When my name is called, I can hear my family cheering and notice my mother wiping tears from her face. I step up on the stage and proudly accept my diploma. I sense that something may fall on my head, as this all seems too good to be true.

Ken and I are en route to the graduation celebration at a hall. I have this strange feeling that an accident may occur en route. I whisper a prayer and then pass my gut feeling off as post stress from the graduation ceremony. However, when we drive around a corner near the hall, we notice that the car my mother and some friends are passengers in . . . has been smashed up, and is stopped in the intersection. A hit and run has just occurred. I enter into a shock mode before discovering that nobody in the car had been injured.

We all enter the hall and celebrate. A party is underway. Family and friends are singing, dancing and eating. I am continually to question: "Can this be really happening?"

The graduation celebration has ended and it is time to commence a teaching career. I start by teaching two on-line courses: Leading From Heart and Mind; and, Spirituality within Leadership, at the University of Calgary. I apply many of the teachings I received when working on my dissertation and when studying Sociology. I start my courses with some of Dale Carnegie's principles. He emphasizes the values of being altruistic and having empathy when working with others. Being genuinely interested in others and showing appreciation and gratitude for their contributions is part of what he encouraged leaders to apply to their credos. He strongly believed that a leader, waiting to be nurtured and cultivated, exists within everyone.

After teaching on line a few years, I apply to teach Sociology courses in the classroom. My first assigned courses involve three classes at the University of Calgary and two courses at Mount Royal College. One Sociology class at the university has four hundred students registered in it. Despite having such a large class, I give students an altruistic assignment, related to the curriculum and the movie *Pay It Forward.* They are to construct social movements to make the world a better place, and then write about their experiences in a paper. I have two teaching assistants when I commence the course. Thus, I trust that together we can mark all the papers and group work. However, as the Christmas holidays are approaching, and the marking is due, one teaching assistant has a car accident. After her accident, I can not locate all the student papers, and I no longer have her to assist me with the marking. And, the other teaching assistant is called back to his home country. Thus, I mark continuously into the morning hours, for at least a week, knowing that when the marks were in, I'd be on a plane to Mexico to celebrate another wedding anniversary.

In Mexico, Ken and I renew our vows on the ocean shore. I wear a long veil that is like a cover up on my white bikini. As our friends, Don and Mohamed walk with me up the beach to meet Ken at an alter facing the ocean, I sing a song I have written for Ken for this special occasion. The waves are whispering a peaceful sound, like a harmony singer. Crowds of people, dressed in bathing suits and drinking tequila gather around us and cheer us on. This is about the fourth time for us to repeat our vows, as we have been renewing them every few years. Thus, I can boast to friends that I have been married a number of times, and then inform them that the marriage is repetitiously to the same man, since high school.

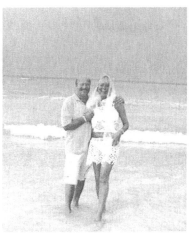

I go to swim with the dolphins the next day. I sense having a spiritual connection. I feel very uplifted before returning to Calgary.

Spring has already set in. It is close to Easter and to my birthday. I have received a Birthday greeting from Kathy that states,

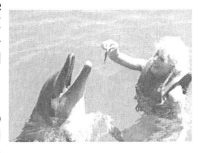

> "Always remember that you are making a major positive difference in people's lives. It's just the way you are. Perhaps it is the sacred energy that is painted in the electromagnetic flashes and wisps and lightening bolts that are projected from you. There is brilliance and vitality in the light you project. You have a bio-electric force that surrounds you. People respond to it consciously and unconsciously seeking your source of higher ener-

gy. Your energy that oscillates at a higher level than most others. You are a link to the sun radiating silently . . . making people feel warm and less threatened by the fragility of life when in your presence."

I treasure her birthday greeting, but I am not sure what she means, as I can never be certain about how others perceive me. However, I am very clear that I am living passionately and that my mission is to make a difference in the world. Kathy may have sensed my intentions, when she heard me speak at a conference.

My birthday celebration has just passed. The telephone rings and I hear an excited voice on the end of the receiver, saying: "you've won an award for your dissertation." I assume it is a joke and then I find a message on email, stating the same message. Within a week, I am on a plane to London, Ontario to receive the Greenfield award for the best doctoral dissertation on educational administration completed in Canada that year. I feel very humbled and nervous. I relax while sitting beside a beautiful tree outside of the place at which I will be honored. When I enter the building, I feel sad that I have no relatives or friends to share the honorable experience with. I sit with a man who has travelled to where my brother spent the last days of his life. My acceptance speech is short as I feel like my sense of gratitude is beyond words.

When I arrive home from London, I have another experience to feel grateful for. I have been asked to speak at a conference in Egypt, and Mohamed has agreed to be my translator and to travel with me. Within a few months, I am on a plane en route to see the pyramids and speak about spiritual intelligence at the American University. While walking up the aisles of the plane, I am reflecting again on having lost my dairy en route to the Holy Land. I am wishing it would suddenly appear at one of the airports I arrive at.

Taking a ride in a boat down the Nile River is an amazing experience, but going inside the Pyramids is even more extraordinary. Singing while in the King's chamber is incred-

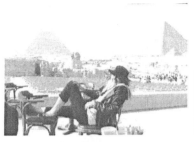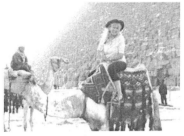

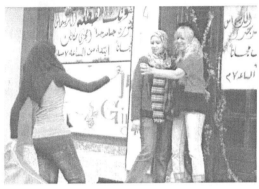

ible, as I feel as if I have a whole symphony choir for my accompaniment. Being inside the pyramids is like stepping inside of an ancient history book. Riding an angry camel is kind of scary. Later, touring the museum augments a further sense of entering into some kind of mysterious world. I appreciate learning about a historical time when people's hearts were weighed after they died. The belief was that if their hearts were as light as feathers, they entered paradise; but, if their hearts were heavy, they entered a dark world. This story reflects some of my research findings, related to heart wisdom.

It is a culture shock to me, being in Egypt. I choose to wear a scarf on my head, in an attempt to better blend in with other females. I fear crossing the streets, as cars speed by without stopping for people crossing the street. Cairo is very crowded and I am bumping into people when walking. I am appreciating the calls to prayer five times a day, which are reminding me to take time to pray. It is very hot and dusty. I have never much spent time in a desert before. But I do recall taking communion, in a desert, with Bishop Henry, in the Holy Land.

I go to the Market close to a huge mosque. I am escorted by a young woman into the mosque. It appears very similar to a church. I feel sacredness, while inside the walls of this building. It is very peaceful when so many people are engaged in prayer.

I am now in a rush to travel home to Calgary to teach a new course that I recently designed. After a week in Egypt, it is challenging to return to the University of Calgary and commence work. I am teaching a course: Leading From Heart and Mind.

When walking down the hallways in the university, I notice a poster advertising that Patch Adams would be speaking in Calgary and I know that I need to find a way to attend his lecture. I recall watching the movie Patch Adams while working on my Masters degree and when battling cancer. I was grateful to learn about the challenges Patch encountered while aiming to bring clowning and laughter into medical school. His experiences have some common ground to me dialoguing about bringing spirituality into education and medicine. His story also reminds me that laughter is the best medicine.

Patch Adams told his audience that he makes a decision every morning to have a great day, and then puts his intention into action. When I spoke with him, after his lecture, he suggested I attend a Re-inventing The Medical Model seminar in Chicago.

Within a few months I am on a plane en route to Chicago, to meet with medical students and doctors interested in inspiring changes in the medical field. After participating in a number of workshops, I join Patch and the group on a clowning venture at a hospital. There, I have an opportunity to observe patients being uplifted by the presence of a group of clowns.

While there, I am reminded of the value of my mother's and sisters' roles as professional clowns at hospitals, festivals and senior homes. They are both amazing clowns, who bring lots of laughter to people. On a few occasions, I attempted to join them, as a fellow clown, but felt like I was very lacking in their talents. Clowning seems to come naturally to them, whereas, I need to really work hard at it.

I am back in the class-room teaching. I am covering a chapter about medical students being socialized. I share Patch Adam's story. He happens to call my cell phone while I am in the classroom, discussing him.

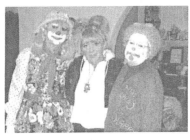

I give the students an opportunity to ask him some questions. They want to know whether or not he really did flash the crowd and medical staff, on his graduation day. He told them, he would just leave them guessing, as the movie is a Hollywood production. They were interested in how he over came "emotional distancing" and "impression management," while working in medicine. He assured them that he truly honors his own authenticity and does it fearlessly.

Before hanging up the phone, Patch asked me if I could attend another Medical conference in the summer. I am tempted to return to Chicago, but I have commitments in Calgary. However, I inform him that I will attend his session in Medicine Hat and then I will drive him to Calgary to catch his plane, before I travel to Thunder Bay.

Reflective question: Can you think of situations where you have experienced "emotional distancing," and or "impression management"? How do you bring humor into your lives?

10

More Challenges, Dancing and Miracles

It is a July first long weekend and I have stepped off Westjet in Thunder Bay to visit family and re-connect with friends. My first stop is at a regular stomping ground, Marina Park, overlooking Lake Superior and the Sleeping Giant. It is a very windy day and the sound of "musical sails" reminds me of a song I wrote about this celestial music. After a short walk around the park, I stand beside the Superior shores, where Ken and I had celebrated a special wedding anniversary. We had arrived by boat and were greeted by a town crier and band. As I reflect on the celebration I search the area for silver decorations dropped there years ago.

When in Thunder Bay, I consult with the physician who had conducted surgery on me. I experience flashbacks when he tells me that I have lumps in three areas of my body. Some medical staff work over time to conduct ultrasounds on me. The physician speaks to me about the high possibility of having cancer return and he suggests that I have further medical check ups in Calgary.

Attending the July 1st celebrations at Marina Park distract me from the doctor's medical report. I sing along to familiar songs sung by musicians who have contributed to the sound tracks in my recordings. In the evening, I visit my friend, Bill, who had sung Scarlet Ribbons with me at the hospital, when I was on route to surgery. We laugh about memories of other patients assuming that I had been heavily medicated, when I was singing.

I also put information given about my health situation aside, as I engage into the joyful spirit of the Calgary stampede and teaching a summer "Leading with Heart and

Mind" course. During the Leadership Institute on campus at the University of Calgary, I engage in a presentation about nurturing "spiritual intelligence." My classroom is filled with students from across the country. I apply humor when sharing stories about the rewards and consequences of trying to cultivate spiritual intelligence within the classroom.

Examples of my teaching style shared during my session, include: calling a student test a "celebration of learning," creating community within the classroom, and honoring students with positive affirmations. A few students who attend this presentation are registered in my "Spirituality Within Leadership" on-line course. On the first evening of this course, during an Elluminate session, three students say that they are cancer survivors. I question whether or not this is some kind of coincidence, associated with my current health issue.

After experiencing additional signs of having a medical issue, I seek consultation with both traditional and alternative medical specialists in Calgary. I am informed that I may have a bit of a "spiritual ego" and I am reminded that even avatars have been known to die of cancer. My medical consultants highly recommended I take a number of tests, including blood and X-rays. I am preparing for a trip to Newport and would rather invest my time into shopping, than focussing on medical issues. I am getting flashbacks of the first time I was diagnosed with cancer, when I was in Newport.

A call from a student conducting research on cancer survivors assists me to see some of the purpose in my pain and health challenges. This student questions me about "congruence" and later forwards me a transcribed version:

> Congruence means living a life of service to others made possible by self-appreciation and self-worth that expresses in healthy boundaries, assertiveness, giving and receiving relationships, and self-care. Scripts, roles and masks are abandoned in favor of unique, personal expression, honesty and clear communication. As a consequence one feels whole, experiences peace and har-

mony within and in relationships, and has a personal relationship/communion with a higher power. Values and beliefs are unique to self and are derived from introspection and meditation. One becomes the author of one's life, priorities and definition of self. One experiences self as a spiritual being and lives in honor of one's own vision, mission, meaning and purpose.

The experience of congruence means living a life of self-esteem, self-respect and recognition of self as important and worthy of self-care. Personal truth is communicated clearly, assertively and without guilt. Habitual thoughts and feelings about self, derived from early socialization processes, 'oughts' and 'shoulds' are abandoned in favor of a sense of personal power and agency to take control of one's life according to inner direction, personal values and beliefs as well as a unique sense of mission in life. One takes care of self due to a sense of self-worth and for the purpose of being able to do what one is intended to do and to render service to others. The key words are choice, being in charge and having control.

I am who I am, I speak my truth, I express my needs, I give of myself on my own terms. I have been, blessed with Irish-Aboriginal roots and have came from a small town environment. My Irish-Aboriginal background afforded me the advantage of growing up in a cultural context enriched by a profound spirituality. Being a spiritual spark that currently inhabits a human body has become part of my nature. I knew with crystal clarity from the moment of being diagnosed with cancer that, although I needed to undergo and adhere to a medical regimen, my spirituality would be my major strength. Experiencing myself as a spiritual being from childhood was difficult to deal with, since it sometimes invited criticism, ridicule and exclusion. I used the cancer experience as one turning point for a major transformation of self. My illness was a wellness. We experience negatives so we can experience positives; negatives and positives are just different sides of the same coin. Because I know grief, I choose joy. "I choose to enjoy chocolate, music, trees, birds, cats, and working with and for people. Seeing everything holistically reverberates through my life journey and extends to my continuous healing journey. In response to suspected cancer recurrences, I re-evaluated my life, changed some priorities and began to create a life of greater inner harmony, less stress and more joy. Although I attribute my survival to many factors, I firmly believe that this is the approach I need to continue on my healing journey

A few months after this interview, I am back at the clinic receiving an ultra sound to check out my health situation. I am anticipating feedback affirming that I am well. But, I am struggling with the news that one of mine and Ken's best friends, Mohamed, will be moving over seas. After hearing the news, I feel as if I am kicking into grief. My heart relives the loss of my brother. After my brother left, and said he'd return within two years, but I never saw him again. I am struggling at the thought of one of my healing team members and dance partners being so far away, while I am facing another health challenge. He promises to return in two years.

To help me cope with my health situation and a friend leaving the city, I sign up for a new dance class, close to the university. I am grateful to discover that both Clay and John, who I dance with on occasion, share a passion for playing the guitar. We get together sometimes, to share our joy of music and dance. I attend the Saturday dance class, after teaching Mass Communications at the university. Thus, I have skipped the introductory dance course scheduled another day. Perhaps this is why I tend to trip on occasion, and an instructor has commented about my lack of muscle memory for certain dance steps. I am attempting to dance a level higher than I have been prepared for. I argue that I dance as if nobody is looking, so being out of step should not be an issue. I stay in the class, and persistently practice, until I learn the steps. Dancing helps me to keep well and I am practicing some dancing, before going to Newport.

After receiving follow up medical examinations, a week before holidays, I head to a shopping mall to pick up vintage clothing for the upcoming Newport trip. I alter my focus from health issues to reflecting on being very close to the ocean. I have a sense of wellness, while anticipating dancing in the Newport Mansions and spending time by the ocean in Corey's Lane.

I step on an Air Canada flight on an early Saturday morning in August and anticipate experiencing an outstanding week of dance and healing. While on the plane, I experience flashbacks of having lost my dairy on a flight, a number of years ago. I am wondering if it is currently in someone's possession, or if there is a very slight possibility that someday, it will arrive in my mail box.

When In Boston, I spend an evening dining with Sr. Audrey, Ken's aunt. I tell her the story of losing my diary on route to the Holy Land. I inform her that I am currently studying to be an associate Sister, in Calgary. She recalls telling me that if she had met me before Ken, I probably would already be part of the Sisterhood. I tell her that I have now entered the formation program in preparation for becoming a Companion in Mission for the Society Sisters Faithful Companions of Jesus.

After praying in the country church Sunday morning, I set out for Newport with Ken. The oceanic scenery on route stirs up a sense of miracle mindedness and living in the moment. I tune into a radio station playing songs from the 60s and 70s. I travel down memory lane of days of singing Elvis and Beatle tunes with my late brother Bob.

Arriving in Newport gives me a warm fuzzy feeling in my stomach. My eyes became glued on the ocean and mansions along the shores. The sun is shining and the temperature is very hot. We head towards Cory's Lane which is about a twenty minute drive from Newport. I am ready to put on my dancing shoes and enter into the rhythm. As we head towards the Vintage registration building, I see familiar faces of dancers from previous years. I am feeling very excited, like a child, just entering Disney World.

We are savoring the light of the moon. I am dressed like a Cinderella, and awaiting Ken to sign my dance card. I look up at the heavens and ask God, if this can this really be me, back here dancing years after having received my first cancer diagnosis.

Suddenly, I hear my song I wrote in Newport called "Savor the light of the moon," playing on the sound system. The dance floor is packed with couples embracing one another. Ken is almost smothering me, as we waltz to the rhythm of my song, in the moonlight. I am weeping, while feeling as if I am experiencing being in heaven, on earth. I question whether or not . . . what I am experiencing can really be real. It appears like just yesterday, I wrote this song, before rushing back to Thunder Bay. Now, years later, from the speakers, I here my own voice singing: She just wants to keep dancing, at the Newport Mansion

> waltz gracefully across the room,
> savor the light of   the moon
> Be queen of the ball,
> in Beechwood hall
> Step into a dream land,
> never let go of his hand.
>
> She's Cinderella tonight,
> all dressed in white
> A long gown and slippers make it right
> Couples dance beside her,
> they seem like a blur
> She's in her own space,
> with a smile on her face

Is this is really happening to me, I keep asking myself. I am a doctor now, alive and well, actually dancing and singing years after receiving a telephone call here in Newport suggesting that my life may be on the line; . . . a telephone call that once challenged my aspirations of ever studying to become a doctor.

Like I wrote in my diary, I recall flying high and then landing low years ago. I had been anticipating a week of carefree travel and then, a simple phone message, suggesting I had cancer, changed my world dramatically, like Cinderella's coach turning back into a pumpkin.

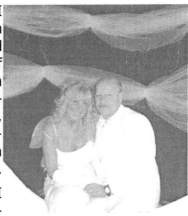

When reflecting back, I recall some humorous memories of travelling on a plane at that time. I was dressed like Cinderella, and thus, received the royal treatment. It was probably assumed by stewardesses that Ken and I had just taken our wedding vows, and were on our honey moon. We were given complimentary wine and snacks.

When we arrived in Thunder Bay, we attended a friend's wedding. During her celebration, I was requested to sing: "My Heart Goes On." The following day, I sensed that my heart was going on and on . . . at Newport; and, I imagined my feet continuously dancing there. But, the reality was . . . I was in a hospital, awaiting emergency surgery. Laughing and singing and praying en route to the operating room enabled me to re-live my wonderful experience of savoring the light of the moon, while I was in a Cinderella role, waltzing at a Newport mansion.

Years later, I am now back in Newport, receiving a message from a clinic, that I will not require surgery. Miraculously, whatever lumps had previously been spotted in a ultra sound, no longer exist. The physician who had scheduled my surgery says that he has no explanation for the positive change in my health. He cancels my surgery and advises me to continue whatever I have been doing to keep healthy.

I am continuing to dance, sing, learn and teach. I am exercising daily, eating nutritious foods, taking Isagenix vitamins, and communing with nature. I am living passion-ately and compassionately one day at a time. I am feeling grateful for all my blessings.

I feel thankful for having just heard an extraordinary lec-ture by, Dr. James Gordon, a pioneer in integrative medi-cine. His address offers practical ways to climb out of the dark psychological dungeon of depression. He believes that depression is not an end point or a disease over which we have no control. It is a sign that our lives are out of balance and that we're stuck.

While using dramatic and inspiring examples from the patients he has worked with over the years, Dr. Gordon explained the practical, mood–healing benefits of: food and nutritional supplements; Chinese medicine; movement, exercise and dance; psychotherapy, meditation and guided imagery; and spiritual practice and prayer. He stresses that depression can be a wake–up call that starts a journey that can help us become whole and happy and one that can change and transform our lives.

To demonstrate some of what he spoke about, Dr. Gordon asked the crowd to shut their eyes, and dance to the upbeat music he had put on the sound system. Within seconds, a room, filled with mainly scholars and health care professionals, appears to be converted into a youthful dance venue. The crowd seems to trust that a suggestion to dance, coming from a medical doctor, must carry credi-bility. Thus, people become submissive and dance coura-geously and joyously.

After the exercise, Dr. Gordon emphasizes that we are social beings, in need of having connection with one anoth-er and healthy role models. Rugged individualism and attempting to make it on our own does not keep us healthy, he insists. We need to return to living everyday joyously, courageously and consciously with ourselves and others.

When people in the audience are questioned how they feel after dancing, they claim they have been uplifted in some way. As a participant and observer, I notice how the majority of people in the audience are smiling, after having danced.

After hearing the lecture, I am inspired to go dancing at Ranchmans. I take a lesson there, in double shuffle. Then, I finish writing a song called "The Dance will never End:

A dance will never end...
When a dance is with a friend
They'll sway across the floor...
And others they'll ignore

The time is always right
Morning afternoon or night..
To be there for a friend..
Their dance will never end

A prayer will never end
When a prayer is with a friend.
God lets them remain as one
Their dance has just begun

Hearts in a sacred dance
Are taking a major chance
Believing that their love
Is Blessed from God above

A dance has just begun,
When Friends are haven fun
Laughing the night away
Then greeting a brand new day!!

I feel joyful after dancing, writing and singing. When I arrive home from Ranchmans, I notice I have a parcel card for a package from a foreign country. I am wondering if my long-lost diary has been found, and has miraculously been sent back to me. Throughout the night, I imagine receiving my sacred dairy, with a note from somebody who has read it. I go to sleep, thinking about things I had written, in it. Then, I fall asleep and dream about being back in Egypt. I am in a museum looking at a mummy that seems to have my face, and is peering up at me. I ask her to return my dairy, and then suddenly I awaken and realize I have only been dreaming.

The dream flashes through my mind during my workday, and when I go to hear Fr. Larre speak about miracles. He talks about having witnessed people being healed, after they had been prayed for. He presents two major cases, where he had been informed by doctors that there was no hope for these individuals to ever be healed from their chronic health conditions. However, the two individuals he mentioned are currently alive and well. One woman, he referred to, had gone to Lourdes to pray, when she was in a wheel chair and could not walk. After praying there, and being prayed for by others, she left her wheel chair at Lourdes, and has been walking ever since. Fr. Larre encouraged us to visit the two individuals he spoke about, in their work places, to see for ourselves how they presently exude health.

I am reminded that in 2001, at a Spirituality in Medicine conference, Dr. David Larson, from the National Institute for Healthcare research, had said that eighty percent of patients believe spiritual faith can help them recover from illnesses; sixty percent believe doctors should address spiritual health and forty percent of patients claim faith is the most important factor in healing from an illness. He spoke about the commonality of people turning to prayer, when they experience chronic illnesses.

Fr Larre spoke about documented physical cures having taken place at Lourdes, which have been considered miracles by the Catholic church. He says the Vatican has applied a scientific method in its observation and proof of physical cures, when determining whether a cure can be considered miraculous.

Perhaps miracles are evidence of themselves. Maybe, we just require and an old heart and child's eyes to recognize them.

Reflective question: Have you observed any miracles in your life or somebody else's life? What did they teach you?